Coronavirus
SCANDAL
EXPOSED

NOT a Conspiracy Theory

DR. JOSHUA PROPHET

CONTENTS

PREFACE

I am exercising my First Amendment rights. There are many among us who are striving to undo the First Amendment for apparent reasons as discussed herein. Most people do not like to be lied to, and I am telling you and showing you how you have been lied to multiple times on this topic. BAMBOOZLED, in fact. Here is an important step for you to take even before you read ALL of this content. "PRESS PAUSE" on whatever you think or believe and look at all of the facts and true information that I have gathered for you. That is what this is, a compilation. Many others have written and voiced their opinions on various topics within. THIS is the most comprehensive accumulation of information on the topic. Please take time to thoughtfully consider the information as it involves: your news and social media exposure, what doctors you trust with your most valuable asset, your health, your wealth, and even your politics. I hope that we have all learned that our vote and our politics absolutely DO matter as we see our great nation crumbling before our very eyes. Then, urge others to purchase their copy and tell others. Please!

Follow us on Twitter @COVIDscaminfo

COVID Awareness Quiz

1. Is the coronavirus (SARS-CoV-2) naturally occurring? Y/N

2. Is the COVID test (PCR) accurate? Y/N

3. Do masks work well to protect from COVID? Y/N

4. Has the # of cases and hospitalizations and deaths been accurately and properly reported? Y/N

5. Was the COVID vaccine properly approved by the FDA and is it effective? Y/N

6. Is Dr Fauci a legit and caring doctor? Y/N

7. Did Biden/Harris fairly win the 2020 election? Y/N
   KEY: ALL NO

If this bothers you, and it SHOULD, then you should read more in

www.coronavirusscandalexposed.com

Then, share this Quiz or our flyer (available for FREE on our website) with as many people as you can.

You knew some things about this weren't quite right. Here is a very complete explanation.

It is a compilation of information on this.

Learn the truth!

Follow us on Twitter @COVIDscaminfo

Coronavirus Scandal Exposed Flyer:

LEARN THE TRUTH!

Press pause. First, you must "press pause" on what you think and believe on the subject and consider this information.

You have been lied to, big time!

Why did Dr. Fauci lie to us???

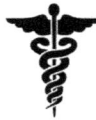

Are COVID tests (PCR) accurate?

Did >500,000 Americans really die from COVID-19? Is it that lethal?

What is the media's role in all of this?

What is the BEST treatment for COVID-19?

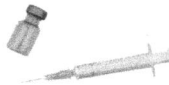

If you have been vaccinated, are you safe?

You have been bamboozled!

Unless you want to start paying taxes to China, become a real Patriot...

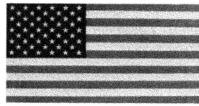

Also included is the downloadable flyer so you can get involved in the "grassroots effort".

Visit our website: coronavirusscandalexposed.com

Follow us on Twitter @COVIDscaminfo

1.

2016 U.S. PRESIDENTIAL ELECTION

We have to start here because this is a very political virus if you have studied it. Hillary Clinton, former Secretary of State ran along with Tim Kaine, former US Senator from Virginia on the Democratic ticket against businessman and "Washington Outsider" Donald Trump along with Mike Pence, former Governor of Indiana on the Republican ticket. Many, including the pollsters predicted that Hillary was going to win, but she lost badly. The Electoral College vote count was 304 for Trump and 227 for Hillary. This upset the Left , including the mainstream media.

The socialist democrats had to wait at least another 4 years to continue their ruinous policies that are destroying America.

2.

RUSSIAN COLLUSION HOAX

So, the Democrats and the mainstream media collectively known as "the Left" went to work to discredit President Trump for his accomplishment of beating Hillary in the election.

Perspective: Hillary Clinton was the Secretary of State during the Obama Administration when economic sanctions were imposed on Russia. Vladimir Putin, the leader of Russia, favored Trump over Hillary at the time. The Russians did interfere with the election by using social media to spread negative information on her. To what extent and what impact it had on the voting is impossible to count.

POLITICS IS DIRTY BUSINESS, BUT THIS LOOKS LIKE POOR SPORTSMANSHIP BY THE DEMOCRATS

The investigation was code named "Crossfire Hurricane" and it began in July 2016 which was prior to the election.

Hillary got involved by paying Christopher Steele, a British Intelligence officer, for the infamous Steele Dosier which tried to incriminate Trump. Then, there were faulty FISA warrants and it snowballed from there.

NBC News - March 24, 2019

> "Special counsel Robert Mueller found no proof that President Donald Trump criminally colluded with Russia and reached no conclusion about whether Trump obstructed justice, Attorney General William Barr told Congress on Sunday, while also announcing that he found insufficient evidence to pursue the matter further."

Here are some resources that give it a different spin than the media gave it:

"The Russia Hoax" by Gregg Jarrett (book)
"The Plot Against the President" by Lee Smith (book)
And a documentary by the same name was created (film).

More Perspective: Honestly, this is just to discredit Hillary Clinton and the Demoncrats further...

Look up her mishandling and lying about the Benghazi Embassy attack. Also, a reminder of her improper use of her personal computer and privileged, Top Secret files that endangered our national security as she was the Secretary of State. Ask why that went unpunished.

3.

BOGUS IMPEACHMENT ATTEMPT OF PRESIDENT TRUMP

From Wikipedia

"The inquiry process which preceded the first impeachment of Donald Trump, 45th president of the United States, was initiated by House Speaker Nancy Pelosi on September 24, 2019,[1] after a whistleblower alleged that Donald Trump may have abused the power of the presidency. **Trump was accused of withholding military aid** as a means of pressuring newly elected president of Ukraine Volodymyr Zelensky to pursue investigations of Joe Biden and his son Hunter[a] and to investigate a conspiracy theory that Ukraine, not Russia, was behind interference in the 2016 presidential election.[3] More than a week after Trump had put a hold on the previously approved aid,[4][b] he made these requests in a July 25 phone call with the Ukrainian president,[6] which the whistleblower said was intended to help Trump's reelection bid.[3]

Believing critical military aid would be revoked, Zelensky made plans to announce investigations into the Bidens on the September 13 episode of CNN's Fareed Zakaria GPS.[5] After Trump was told of the whistleblower complaint in late August[7] and elements of the events had begun to leak, the aid was released on September 11 and the planned interview was cancelled.[5] Trump declassified a non-verbatim summary of the call on September 24,[6][8] the day the impeachment inquiry began. The whistleblower's complaint was given to Congress the following day and subsequently released to the public.[9] The White House corroborated several of the allegations, including that a record of the call between Trump and Zelensky had been stored in a highly restricted system in the White House normally reserved for classified information.[10][11]

In October, three congressional committees (Intelligence, Oversight, and Foreign Affairs) deposed witnesses including Ukraine ambassador Bill Taylor,[12] Laura Cooper (the top Pentagon official overseeing Ukraine-related U.S. policy),[13] and former White House official Fiona Hill.[14] Witnesses testified that they believed Trump wanted Zelensky to publicly announce investigations into the Bidens and Burisma (a Ukrainian natural gas company on whose board Hunter Biden had served)[5][15] and 2016 election interference.[16] On October 8, in a letter from White House Counsel Pat Cipollone to House Speaker Pelosi, the White House officially responded that it would not cooperate with the investigation due to concerns including that there had not yet been a vote of the full House of Representatives and that interviews of witnesses were being conducted privately. [17][18] On October 17, White House acting chief of staff Mick Mulvaney responded to a reporter's allegation of quid pro quo saying: "We do that all the time with foreign policy. Get over it." He walked back his comments later, asserting that there had been "absolutely no quid pro quo" and that Trump had withheld military aid to Ukraine over concerns of the country's corruption. [19][20]"

This, again, is just dirty politics. They had no reason to investigate President Trump. They should be investigating the Bidens as Hunter Biden, son of Joe Biden has been found to be suspiciously funneling millions of dollars from Ukraine and specifically the natural gas company, Burisma. See also the Hunter Biden laptop story. Did you know that Hunter Biden has zero knowledge or experience in this field, yet they put him on the Board...In Ukraine...No jobs in US??? The timing of this is interesting. The media buries the Hunter Biden story, yet falsely accuses the President of the United States. Also, note that the timing is going into the election and puts a false smudge on the President.

Please watch the FoxNews (Tucker Carlson) interview of Tony Bobulinski, former business partner of the Bidens. Also, watch videos of laptop repairman, John Paul MacIsaac. So, Hunter spilled water or some other fluid on his laptop causing damage to it, so he took it to the computer repair shop, left it there over 90 days and then it legally became the property of the repair shop. You should see what is on there. It is very incriminating, but the

FBI buried the story because they are owned by the leftists. This story being released and covered properly by the media likely would have caused Biden not to gain the White House.

Go to www.hannity.com/media-room/ Trump-administration-accomplishments

- Almost 4 million jobs created since the election.

- More Americans are now employed than ever recorded before in our history.

- We have created more than 400,000 manufacturing jobs since my election.

- Manufacturing jobs growing at the fastest rate in more than **THREE DECADES**.

- Economic growth last quarter hit 4.2 percent.

- New unemployment claims recently hit a 49-year low.

- Median household income has hit the highest level ever recorded.

- African-American unemployment has recently achieved the lowest rate ever recorded.

- Hispanic-American unemployment is at the lowest rate ever recorded.

- Asian-American unemployment recently achieved the lowest rate ever recorded.

- Women's unemployment recently reached the lowest rate in 65 years.

- Youth unemployment has recently hit the lowest rate in nearly half a century.

- Lowest unemployment rate ever recorded for Americans without a high school diploma.

- Under my Administration, veterans' unemployment recently reached its lowest rate in nearly 20 years.

- Almost 3.9 million Americans have been lifted off food stamps since the election.

- The Pledge to America's Workers has resulted in employers committing to train more than 4 million Americans. We are committed to VOCATIONAL education.

- 95 percent of U.S. manufacturers are optimistic about the future—the highest ever.

- Retail sales surged last month, up another 6 percent over last year.

- Signed the biggest package of tax cuts and reforms in history. After tax cuts, over $300 billion poured back in to the U.S. in the first quarter alone.

- As a result of our tax bill, small businesses will have the lowest top marginal tax rate in more than 80 years.

- Helped win U.S. bid for the 2028 Summer Olympics in Los Angeles.

- Helped win U.S.-Mexico-Canada's united bid for 2026 World Cup.

- Opened ANWR and approved Keystone XL and Dakota Access Pipelines.

- Record number of regulations eliminated.

- Enacted regulatory relief for community banks and credit unions.

- Obamacare individual mandate penalty GONE.

- My Administration is providing more affordable healthcare options for Americans through association health plans and short-term duration plans.

- Last month, the FDA approved more affordable generic drugs than ever before in history. And thanks to our efforts, many drug companies are freezing or reversing planned price increases.

- We reformed the Medicare program to stop hospitals from overcharging low-income seniors on their drugs— saving seniors hundreds of millions of dollars this year alone.

- Signed Right-To-Try legislation.

- Secured $6 billion in NEW funding to fight the opioid epidemic.

- We have reduced high-dose opioid prescriptions by 16 percent during my first year in office.

- Signed VA Choice Act and VA Accountability Act, expanded VA telehealth services, walk-in-clinics, and same-day urgent primary and mental health care.

- Increased our coal exports by 60 percent; U.S. oil production recently reached all-time high.

- United States is a net natural gas exporter for the first time since 1957.

- Withdrew the United States from the job-killing Paris Climate Accord.
- Cancelled the illegal, anti-coal, so-called Clean Power Plan.
- Secured record $700 billion in military funding; $716 billion next year.
- NATO allies are spending $69 billion more on defense since 2016.
- Process has begun to make the Space Force the 6th branch of the Armed Forces.
- Confirmed more circuit court judges than any other new administration.
- Confirmed Supreme Court Justice Neil Gorsuch and nominated Judge Brett Kavanaugh.
- Withdrew from the horrible, one-sided Iran Deal.
- Moved U.S. Embassy to Jerusalem.
- Protecting Americans from terrorists with the Travel Ban, upheld by Supreme Court.
- Issued Executive Order to keep open Guantanamo Bay.
- Concluded a historic U.S.-Mexico Trade Deal to replace NAFTA. And negotiations with Canada are underway as we speak.
- Reached a breakthrough agreement with the E.U. to increase U.S. exports.
- Imposed tariffs on foreign steel and aluminum to protect our national security.

- Imposed tariffs on China in response to China's forced technology transfer, intellectual property theft, and their chronically abusive trade practices.

- Net exports are on track to increase by $59 billion this year.

- Improved vetting and screening for refugees, and switched focus to overseas resettlement.

- We have begun BUILDING THE WALL. Republicans want STRONG BORDERS and NO CRIME. Democrats want OPEN BORDERS which equals MASSIVE CRIME.

That was posted 10-16-2018.

Also, please try to take an objective view of what President Trump accomplished. Our economy was the best ever, unemployment was at record low rates (with more African Americans employed than during Obama)and look at GDP and GNP figures.

President Trump had done nothing worthy of Impeachment charges and he was found to be not guilty.

Impeachment failed…release the virus…

4.

CORONAVIRUS UNLEASHED

First, let's talk about germs. The two that you hear the most about are bacteria and viruses. Bacteria have cell walls and viruses do not. Most anti-bacterials and hand sanitizers work by breaking down the cell wall of the bacteria. They don't work well on viruses, but don't feel bad. Somebody just made a bunch of money on that misinformation. Viruses come in two main types: DNA and RNA. The messenger RNA type is unique and troublesome. Viruses may have a protein coat called a capsid and the coronavirus has these unique and also troublesome spike proteins. A virus may have an envelope made of lipid (fat). In order to replicate/multiply, a virus requires a host, that is a living being with cells that it may attack and multiply itself. It is very difficult to really know how long a virus can live outside of a host.

The name of this virus is SARS-CoV-2 (Severe Acute Respiratory Syndrome Coronavirus 2) and the name of the disease condition it causes is called COVID-19 (Coronavirus Infectious Disease 2019) That is, it was created with American funding that Dr Fauci relayed there via EcoHealth Alliance even though this "gain of function" research had been banned by the US government. It was released from the Wuhan Institute of Virology (man-made) and NOT from the wet market as the narrative went. That was a BIG lie propagated by the liberal media! I have proof, read on...

Symptoms of COVID-19 (from Wikipedia)

"Symptoms of COVID-19 are variable, ranging from mild symptoms to severe illness. Common symptoms include headache, loss of smell and taste, nasal congestion and runny nose, cough, muscle pain, sore throat, fever, diarrhea, and breathing difficulties. People with the same infection may have different symptoms, and their symptoms may change over time. Three common clusters of symptoms have been identified: one respiratory symptom cluster with cough, sputum, shortness of breath, and fever; a musculoskeletal symptom cluster with muscle and joint pain, headache, and fatigue; a cluster of digestive symptoms with abdominal pain, vomiting, and diarrhea. In people without prior ear, nose, and throat disorders, loss of taste combined with loss of smell is associated with COVID-19."

Let's talk more about the origin of this coronavirus. THE CORONAVIRUS WAS DEFINITELY CREATED SYNTHETICALLY BY HUMANS IN THE WUHAN INSTITUTE OF VIROLOGY IN CHINA. Whether it was released accidently or intentionally is now being debated, but IF you read this document carefully you may draw the conclusion that this was all planned. (Be sure to research the past actions of Mr. Bill Gates)

So, why did Dr. Fauci lie to us. He told us through the lying media that it was naturally occurring. He claims to be a "scientist". What is the probability of it being naturally occurring? NIL! Now that his emails have surfaced, we see that he did know it was "Gain of function" research. That is when you take a virus and supercharge it to damage humans even more. 'Bioweapon' is another word. Fauci knew all about it because he funded it with US dollars. So, he had a bit of a reason to deny the truth. Now, various politicians (such as Rep. Jim Jordan, OH and Rand Paul, MD from KY) and people in the media are calling for an investigation and so forth…Well, that is seemingly the normal thing to do. You are not likely to just walk into the lab 18 months later and find what you are looking for. Get it? The circumstantial evidence, the law of probability against zoonosis of the coronavirus and the content of the "Fauci emails" are adequate proof to indict.

Do you think it is a mere coincidence that the architect of the virus, Ralph Baric, PhD. , UNC-CH had previously collaborated on virus research with "The Bat Lady", Zhengli Shi, a key researcher at the Wuhan Institute of Virology? I have seen the research papers. Also, after multiple workers at the Wuhan lab got sick, they scrubbed any record of it.

Did you know that it has a ~99% survival rate?

This is the key evidence that the lockdowns should not have happened, but they are just a part of the bigger agenda.

To give you a bit of perspective, my friend told me in March of 2020 that the Democrats were going to use the coronavirus lockdowns to impact the 2020 Presidential Elections in their favor. I thought it was bizarre. It happened!

Be sure to read the article that somehow got printed in Newsweek on 04/28/2020 by Fred Guterl entitled "Dr. Fauci Backed Wuhan Lab with U.S. Dollars for Risky Coronavirus Research". This lab leak theory got squashed along with the best ways to treat it.

There is a video I want you to watch also. It is called "Plandemic". A friend shared it with me in May of 2020. It has been very difficult for me to watch things unfold knowing what I know. This video got banned by YouTube. Now, we have to address the issue of censorship. The normal human being initially assumes something must be wrong or dishonest about this video. Perhaps it is indeed the "fact checkers" who ARE the perpetrators. Note that YouTube is owned by Google and in case you haven't heard "Big Tech" is totally involved with all of this. So, when a video gets banned, where do you go to watch it? www.brighteon.com

Take note of that.

Here is a FB post from March 30, 2020

> "The Wuhan Lab is the house that Fauci built. Don't let this fake narrative out there distract from the incestuous relationship between the US and the WHO and CCP money. The spin is dizzying."
>
> -a conspiracy theorist

There was another video interviewing a very prominent MD named Dr Lee Merritt

She stated that the coronavirus IS highly contagious (because it is new) but it is benign, that is non-lethal. The spike proteins make it more dangerous. The initial virus was more lethal, but there is a 99% survival rate. Compare to Ebola and HIV, which had approximately a 10% survival rate, which was a death sentence.

Let me say that again as you recall the paranoia invoked by the media. It has an approx. 99% survival rate! This is very close to the flu and they never made us wear masks and lockdown for the flu in spite of recent surges.

She does not recommend a vaccine for this. Rather she states that the therapeutics work quite well, including medications Ivermectin and Hydroxichloroquine . She also recommends vitamin D, quercitin and zinc. Many other doctors also recommend vitamin C and other supplements to stimulate immune function, but this also got squashed as useless. Could it be that if you can not get a patent on it then it has no value to some??? Also, curiously the 2 plants that make Hydrochloroquine recently burned down. This is beginning to stink. Speaking of stinky animals, they just skipped that normal step in testing a vaccine because they knew it would kill the animals as prior mRNA vaccine trials have.

The SARS-CoV-2 virus particularly endangers certain people and those with certain health conditions: the elderly, obesity, diabetics, immune suppressed, cardiovascular disease and others. These are what we call comorbidities. They are other health conditions that could lead to death. The fatality rate ranges from .02 to .4%, which is comparable to the seasonal flu. So, why did this virus get such attention? Was it because it was an election year? Was it part of a grander plan? Read on.

One big reason for the mass hysteria early on was the prediction of British "scientist", Professor Neil Ferguson of Imperial College in London that over 500,000 in the United Kingdom and 2 million in the United States. This same individual had made grave predictions in the past about fatalities caused by mad cow disease and avian flu. He was badly wrong each time, so why should we have trusted him?

The origin of the virus is a huge question. Politicians and reporters will always say that we need to investigate this. During President Trump's administration, Secretary of State, Mike Pompeo tried to conduct an investigation into the source of the virus, but it got squashed by the bad guys. It is appalling to me that the lab leak theory would be disregarded and discredited. There is a back story. President Biden sent a team to the Wuhan Institute of Virology tasked to investigate the origins of the virus. Peter Daszak, head of EcoHealth Alliance, was ON the task force. Wake up, reader! He was involved with creating the virus. Of course, his report is going to say that there is nothing to see here. Be sure to view the You Tube video from 2015 where he states that coronaviruses are easy to manipulate.

Here is some of the science behind the origin of SARS-CoV-2 virus. It was previously known to infect bats and not humans. The process called zoonosis is when the virus "learns" how to infect humans. For that to happen naturally (as in at a wet market as Fauci has tried to tell us) has a probability of approximately zero chance. It's not just a coincidence that the Wuhan Institute of Virology is right there and Dr Fauci funded the "gain of function" research on this particular virus. That has all come to light, but it's disgusting how long it has been delayed.

 Dr Fauci is holding a smoking gun AND the ballistics match too.

06-16-2021 video surfaced (4:20 min.)

Gravitas: The Interview China Tried to Hide Wuhan Coronavirus. Dr. Ai Fen was a doctor at the hospital in Wuhan and she saw some of the first COVID patients. She has disappeared.

Consider this! Patents for the virus SARSCoV2 were issued PRIOR to the COVID outbreak. Big Money! Let's investigate that along with the vaccine patents. See David Martin videos.

5.

CORONAVIRUS TESTING

First, let me make brief mention of antibody testing as it is of little value because the body produces the antibodies to the virus after approximately 1-2 weeks and that is too much time for a person to be spreading the infection to others. Dr. Brix mentioned this fact in a press briefing early on in the "pandemic".

The name for the most common test for coronavirus is the PCR Test. It is performed by using a swab to take a sample from the nasopharyngeal areas by sticking it up your nose or down your throat. It really is great fun. Perhaps you should not have it done and here is why. It is NOT accurate and the founder of the test said that it is not for this purpose. It is very important for you to understand the role of the testing in all of this so I will go into some lengthy discussion.

Dr. Kary Mullis, PhD. Was the creator if the PCR (Polymerase Chain Reaction) test and he won the Nobel Prize in Chemistry for it in 1993. He discovered a technique that allows replication of DNA molecules, so it is a method of copying and amplifying DNA. Coronavirus is RNA virus so who knows if even works at all on RNA? That is not the crux of the issue, though. Go back in time to when Dr. Fauci in his same job was battling the AIDS crisis, which is known to be caused by the HIV virus. Back then, Dr. Mullis battled with Dr. Fauci telling him that the test is not for the purpose of diagnosing a specific virus. So, it is upsetting to know that Dr Fauci was absolutely aware of this fact. I will provide more evidence that the test is not accurate for diagnosing if a person has COVID and think of the ramifications.

"Anyone can test positive for practically anything with a PCR test, if you run it long enough…with PCR if you do it well, you can find almost anything in anybody…it does not tell you that you are sick."

-Dr. Kary Mullis, PhD. (creator of the PCR test)

What did he mean by "if you run it long enough?" This is key. The sample is run through a number of cycles or processes in the lab. The WHO (World Health Organization) and possibly the CDC (Center for Disease Control) set the number of cycles to run the specimen through. This is a Facebook quote by Dr David Samadi, MD "PCR test are unreliable due to the amplification threshold. Anything over 17 cycles is worthless. In the USA, we use 35 cycles. The WHO recommends 40-45 cycles. Totally worthless. At that many amplifications you are just picking up the presence of any virus. Useless."

Dr Allen Spreen, MD stated "PCR test is not accurate"

Dr Sherri Tenpenny posted on Parler "THIS IS HUGE!!! A (+) PCR test with count value of 37 or higher (level set by most labs) means the test is a FALSE POSITIVE. No virus can be found or cultured. You are NOT sick. No quarantine. No shutdown. The CASE-DEMIC will be over. Should demand that all labs release their count values."

Dr Carrie Madej, DO posted on Facebook "Of all the positive COVID tests of the 9,000+ students at Cambridge University tested in the week to 6 December, EVERY SINGLE ONE was found to be a False Positive after a second test."

THIS IS HUGE! READ THIS TIMELINE...

www.totalityofevidence.com/pandemic-timeline/pandemic-2020/January13,2020

Even Elon Musk Tweeted on 06/29/2020 "There are a ridiculous number of false positive COVID-19 tests, in some cases ~50%. False positives scale linearly with # of tests. This is a big part of why COVID-19 positive tests are going up while hospitalizations and mortality are declining. Anyone who tests positive should retest."

Here is another quote, author unknown-

The PCR test is the COVID test and it does not test for COVID. The inventor, Kary Mullis, said so. Fauci is using the fake test to tell healthy people that they're sick so they take the poisonous COVID vaccine. Fauci did the same thing in the '80s, using the same faulty PCR test for HIV, so that his uninformed victims would take the fatal AIDS medication called AZT. Fauci is not a doctor, he's a war criminal..."

Please note that Fauci was in favor of medication back then to treat AIDS (Auto Immune Deficiency Syndrome) which is caused by HIV (Human Immunodeficiency Virus). AIDS had just about a 10% survival rate. Now, fast forward to the passing of the Bayh-Dole Act, which made it legal for government officials to obtain patents on inventions arising from research done with federal funding. Suddenly, Fauci has no faith in the medications to work on COVID-19 even though they had been proven to work. He is reported to have ownership in a COVID vaccine patent as does Bill Gates, the computer mogul and billionaire. Surely, I digress. Send the forensic accountants.

Do you find it coincidental that the WHO reduced the number of cycles to be done in the PCR test for COVID just after January 21 when Biden was inaugurated?

Also, do you find it coincidental that Dr Kary Mullis, the founder of the PCR test, died in August of 2019? Go to www.bitchute. com for a 4 minute video "The Mysterious Death of Dr Fauci's Most Notable Critic."

I would like to verify that he died of pneumonia.

Keep reading and put all of the pieces together.

"Flatten the Curve"- This is as good of a place as any to talk about flattening the curve. Dr Fauci used the phrase when he was first asking all of us to wear masks and to social distance, etc… It refers to minimizing the number of fatalities from COVID. News Flash-by June 2020 the curve WAS flattened! {Go to www.cdc.gov/nchs/nvss/vsrr/COVID19/index.htm and view the reported weekly death toll from COVID} But, did he say that it was? NO! At this time the media began to beat us every day with the number of cases that showed up positive on a bogus test. Remember, COVID has a 99% survival rate. We never did all of this when the flu incidence and deaths spiked up in 2017/2018 for example. Not an election year. Maybe Fauci should be sued class action style for not saving those lives lost to the flu. Reverse psychology. Multiple wrongful deaths! Also, be sure to read the AMA's position on masks in the mask section. It all ties together. Keep in mind that the POTUS (President of the United States) is considered to be the most powerful position on earth. The Democrats wanted to force mail in voting because it is easier to cheat that way. Look at what actually happened and not what the mainstream media feeds you. Our democracy and our way of life is at stake. Watch the vote recounts and the class action lawsuit forthcoming.

6.

CORONAVIRUS #CASES AND #DEATHS REPORTING FRAUD

THIS IS HUGE! THIS DISPELS ONE OF THE BIGGEST LIES YOU HAVE BEEN TOLD EVERY DAY (IF YOU WATCH THE LIBERAL MAINSTREAM MEDIA)

The falsely and highly skewed number of cases comes from the gross inaccuracy of the PCR test as discussed above. There is one other devious detail, though. They needed to incentivize the medics to participate in this charade, so they gave them via Medicare or other insurers, I am told, $13,000 per COVID-19 case and they got $39,000 IF the patient went on a ventilator. Did ventilators save lives? I heard that you have an 80% chance of dying once on a ventilator. This is another prime example of attempted medical heroics following the wrong treatment!

The lying liberal media has been telling us that over 500,000 Americans have died from COVID. That is simply not true! Here is how I know. I will apply the Law of Probability as I did in knowing that the virus WAS created in the lab and not at the market as we were falsely told. The CDC website keeps track of how many Americans die each year. First, the good news: approximately 4 million babies are born in America each year resulting in a net population increase. If you go to CDC. gov you can find these charts and tables that show in recent years just under 3 million die in America at a rate of .9% per year. Considering that COVID was a new killer on the scene, using the LAW of Probability, we would project that there would have been almost 3.5 million total deaths in 2020, but there were not. The other causes of death would logically remain relatively constant. In actuality, there was only an increase in the total number of deaths in America going from 2019 to 2020 of approximately 50,000. According to my math, that is a 10X lie the liberal media has been feeding us every day lately. We should have required autopsy reports on each to properly document this. Please forgive the morbidity of all this, but every bit of this comes back to the Demoncrats agenda. There is a big difference in dying from COVID and dying with COVID. Ponder that. Most of these people died from the comorbidity that they had and perhaps they did get infected by the virus also. Big difference. Comorbidities are other health problems the individual had, such as diabetes, heart disease, suppressed immune system and others.

80% of COVID deaths worldwide were obese people. The average age of the person who died from was 80 years of age. In fact, 92% of deaths in the US were over 85 years old and with an average of 2.6 comorbidities. Is it also true that people die every day? Incidentally, the average life expectancy for women in the U.S. is 81 and for men in U.S. it is 77 years.

We will never know exact numbers of COVID fatalities because there is so much fraud around it. The test is not accurate. The diagnosis is not properly made. People die of other reasons and they are labelled "COVID death" for a wrong political agenda. Then, people died from the vaccine and Remdesivir. Should we count those also?

The WHO played a role in this, too. They set the number of cycles for PCR tests high at 45. The WHO, via ICD-10 (International Classification of Disease) formed new diagnosis codes for doctors to use. Initially, there were 2. One basically said that the patient definitely has COVID and the other one said that this kind of looks like COVID, so let's just call it COVID to boost the numbers. I am stating this in the vernacular and with light hearted sarcasm, but it sickens me to think of what they have done and WHY??? The WHO and/or CDC has produced at least 6 other similar diagnosis codes in early 2021.

The 2 initial diagnosis codes for COVID are:

1. U07.1 COVID-19 with virus identified
2. U07.2 COVID-19 presumed- virus not identified

For fatality stats by CDC go to:

www.cdc.gov/nchs/nvss/vsrr/covid_weekly

NCHS=National Center for Health Statistics
NVSS=National Vital Statistics System

Another source: Coronavirus False Alarm

Pages 17, 23, 28, 35

See also: www.NYPost.com/2020/04/07feds-classify-all-coronavirus-patient-deaths-as-covid-19-deaths

Many of you reading this have lost someone to COVID, and I am deeply sorry.

In January 2022, the CDC admitted that only about 50, 000 Americans had died from COVID and not the frightening 836,000 number. (FEARMONGERING)

7.

TREATMENT OF COVID-19 IS DEAD WRONG

This was a post that circulated on Facebook. Did you see it? October 12, 2020-

"BREAKING NEWS: The world renowned experts in their fields, after a 4-day conference regarding COVID-19, declare that WE SHOULD ALL GO BACK TO LIVING NORMALLY, PRACTICING SIMPLE HYGEINE AND STAYING HOME WHEN SICK (NO FACE MASKS OR SOCIAL DISTANCING) and only protect the most vulnerable populations with more protective measures!

From October 1-4, 2020, the American Institute for Economic Research had a remarkable meeting of top epidemiologists, economists, and journalists, to discuss the global emergency created by the unprecedented use of state compulsion in the management of the COVID-19 pandemic. The result is The Great Barrington Declaration, which urges a "Focused Protection" strategy.

Imagine if the known effective treatment strategies were utilized in each case.

Schools and universities should be open for in-person teaching. Extracurricular activities, such as sports, should be resumed. Young, low-risk adults should work normally, rather than from home. Restaurants and other businesses should open. Arts, music, sport and other cultural activities should resume."

These are some of the top minds in the country and in the world who did not have a vested interest in this scandal. It is not reckless. Keep in mind that young people essentially do not die from this. The elderly and high-risk people are advised to be protected and more cautious. Over 34 experts created and signed this. This is from the top MDs and PhDs from the most respected institutions in the world. This was nothing to sneeze at, but Fauci, et al ignored it as they had a mission to fulfill, which you may not fully understand, yet. Keep on digging for the truth. It is in these pages.

The most impressive MD treatment plan I have seen was presented by Dr. Peter McCullough, MD in a video I saw through Dr Mercola's site and/or email newsletter. www.mercola.com is a great source of health information. Dr. McCullough recommends

Monoclonal Antibodies (source Wikipedia-Antibodies made by cloning unique blood cells. All subsequent antibodies derived this way trace back to a unique parent cell." This has been touted as one of the best treatments for COVID. In fact, President Trump had monoclonal antibody therapy when he caught it and he survived. Next, Dr. McCullough recommends the drug Hydrochloroquine and/or Ivermectin and then there are multiple supplements that support immune function, including Vitamin C and D, Zinc, Elderberry, Echinacea, Quercitin, Garlic, and others...

I watched one video of a MD appearing before a U.S. government committee and he was just raving about how effective Ivermectin is. He was ignored by Fauci, et al. due to his agenda.

A Facebook post- "While the World is on a vaccine frenzy, the Indian government is distributing a home COVID kit with Zinc, Doxycycline and Ivermectin. The cost is $2.65 per person.

News Flash(aside)- "India is the country that kicked Bill Gates out. Because his polio vaccine experiments disguised as "charity" have given 500,000 children polio and caused paralysis. We know this because the victims have the strain that is in his vaccine." I believe he also distributed his polio vaccine in Africa via the Bill and Melinda Gates Foundation. Some people say that Gates wants to reduce the world population. Read on...

So, we have plenty of therapeutics that work...

Here is a key piece to the puzzle. For Dr. Fauci to get Emergency Use Authorization for the COVID-19 vaccine one major stipulation was that there had to be no effective therapeutics.

Remember when I told you that when Dr. Fauci was "battling" the AIDS crisis he was all in favor of the drug AZT (which some believe is what killed patients). Remember the Bayh-Dole Act which became law allowing government officials to patent and profit from results of government funded research. Also, keep in mind that the COVID vaccine is messenger RNA vaccine. Do you know how many messenger RNA vaccines of any kind the FDA has approved? How about none? ZERO! The last report I got was that there is normally an animal trial stage before humans, but that got skipped allegedly to rush the vaccine to the public or actually because the animals in prior m-RNA vaccine trials either got very sick or died. Do you see what has been going on?

See also, July 2020 issue of <u>Science</u>, Public Health Policy, and the Law.

See also the Nuremberg Code

See also videos by Dr. Vernon Coleman, MD.

He is an elderly British gentleman who does a very good job of explaining this.

Later in the pandemic, they got the drug, Remdesivir, approved. Look at the study Fauci quotes with Remdesivir treating Ebola virus saying that it is safe and effective. It killed 54% of the people in the study! Also, watch Dr. Bryan Ardis' video on the chemical makeup of the spike proteins on the coronavirus and the similarity to Remdesivir. Ask why are other effective treatments being banned in an otherwise free country???

That video is called "Don't Drink the Water".

8.

MASKS ARE NOT HEALTHY

(Fauci bucks AMA Guidelines for Mask Wearing)

There has been much debate on the subject of mask wearing through the COVID crisis (notice that I did not call it a pandemic here because little did you know that the WHO recently changed their definition of what a pandemic is taking out the requirement that the disease be truly lethal, in effect). Indeed, even Dr Fauci was on record at one point to say that masks do not work. Many believe that they were pushed by the liberals and left wingers in government to have a visible physical manifestation of this situation that would require people to vote by mail, again because it is easier to cheat on the vote count that way. Others think it is all just about control as the liberal radical left wingers attempt to convert the United States of America to a socialist state. I digress intentionally. Consider that in recent years the number of flu deaths spiked up in America. And could that be because a vaccine makes you more likely to get it next time? Why were we not forced to wear masks during the recent upsurge in flu deaths? Was it because it was not an election year? Should Dr Fauci be sued on a class action level for NOT having us wear masks because according to his feigned belief that masks work, he could have saved all of those lives that were lost to the flu during for example 2017 and 2018.

Masks is probably the biggest topic when we are discussing "the science" behind all of this. Look here.

The Journal of the AMA (JAMA), which is a very prestigious and respected journal cited what are or should be the guidelines for mask wearing. Note that the date was April 21, 2020. To summarize, it states that IF an individual is sick and they come in close contact with another, then masks should be worn. It goes on to say that healthy people SHOULD NOT WEAR A MASK to prevent infection. Certainly, Fauci was aware of this, but at that point in time, he did not have the AMA behind him on this scandal. Here is the synopsis.

Journal of the American Medical Association (JAMA); April 21, 2020 Volume 323, Number 15

> "Face masks should be used only by individuals who have symptoms of respiratory infection such as coughing, sneezing, or, in some cases, fever. Face masks should also be worn by healthcare workers, by individuals who are taking care of or are in close contact with people who

have respiratory infections, or otherwise as directed by a doctor. Face masks should NOT be worn by healthy individuals to protect themselves from acquiring respiratory infection because there is no evidence to suggest that face masks worn by healthy individuals are effective in preventing people from becoming ill. Face masks should be reserved for those who need them because masks can be in short supply during periods of widespread infection. Because N95 respirators require special fit testing, they are not recommended for use by the general public."

Some might want to argue that this Coronavirus was somehow different making it an extenuating circumstance. I want to remind you that it has about a 99% survival rate and IF treated properly it would be even less chance of dying. It is worldwide so you really can't feasibly "hide" from it for the rest of your life. Certainly, a mask is a physical barrier to the airways and it may block some germs. But,…

They did another research study on mask effectiveness, but the results did not come out as desired so it did not get published. Hmmm. That is fishy to me. In fact, it was funded by Fauci's NIAID/NIH Grant to researchers at Yale and was going to be published in the British Medical Journal. It was WITHDRAWN! The title was to be "Decrease in Hospitalizations for COVID-19 after Mask Mandates in 1083 US Counties". It was on 11-01-2020. "Abstract-Withdrawal: The authors have withdrawn this manuscript because there are increased rates of SARS-CoV-2 cases in the areas that we originally analyzed in this study. New analyses in the context of the third surge in the United States are therefore needed and will be undertaken directly in conjunction with the creators of the publicly available databases on cases, hospitalizations, testing rates, etc.

Let's go back to "the science" and add a dash of hypocrisy. The major purpose of mandatory mask wearing is to prevent spread from a person who is asymptomatic to another person. Fauci was quoted to say. "There is some asymptomatic transmission. In all the history of respiratory born viruses of any type, asymptomatic transmission has never been the driver of outbreaks..." So, essentially everyone on the planet was forced by government authorities to strap a worthless piece of fabric over their face for many months until they could have their election results skewed to their preference.

Did you know that Dr Fauci is a Democrat? In fact, most of the major players in this scandal are democrats.

Zero in on what is going on in the body when it initially gets infected with a virus. The body wants to recognize foreign invaders via the immune system and get rid of them. The virus' objective for its survival is to get into the hosts cells and specifically to the DNA to multiply itself. It's called replication and it is like mass production of the virus. A fever often initiates a number of days after exposure to the virus. Schools historically send kids home if they have a fever. So, why don't they stick a mask on them and send them home to quarantine until well?

"There is no scientific evidence that symptom-free people without cough or fever spread the disease." Coronavirus: False Alarm? Facts and Figures, by Dr. Sucharit Bhakdi, MD and Dr. Karina Reiss, PhD.

Many people posted on Facebook during the COVID crisis "I have an immune system." This reflects a different perspective on how to manage these pesty infections. The immune system is quite complex, but here is a simple overview. Its main job is to run interference for the cells that make up the body. That is, it must identify what is "self" and "non-self". All of the cells of the body are "self" and any invader, such as a virus, bacteria, other microbe, dust or pollen or otherwise. The T-cells, specialized white blood cells, produced in the thymus gland perform this function. Then the body makes antibodies to help defend against this invader in case it ever decides to come back. There is also a removal process that involves the macrophage cells which work like "Pac-Man" to get rid of these invaders. When you see these intricacies of the human body it takes even greater faith to believe that this just evolved like this. Probability zero!

Did you ever wonder why the medical profession has little interest in strengthening the immune response? Many supplements do strengthen the immune system. Could it be because they can not get a patent on it and charge exorbitant amounts of money like the pharmaceutical industry does? They do, however, give multiple different drugs that actually intentionally weaken the immune system, such as some cancer drugs and drugs for auto-immune diseases. By the way, Dr Fauci has been on record to say that these nasty little spike proteins that he had engineered in the

Wuhan Lab will cause future auto-immune problems. Thanks for that. Also, since the COVID vaccine was forced on us, birth rates in Australia have dropped by 70%! That is a big number. This is crimes against humanity.

This has made me curious if anyone has researched the mechanism of action of the different supplements that we know work to improve immune function and ideally if a literature search has been done on it, and then make it widespread knowledge.

Also, watch the documentary GMO/OMG for info on the rise in auto-immune conditions caused by GMOs.

"Asymptomatic transmission of COVID-19 didn't occur at all, study of 10 million finds-Only 300 asymptomatic cases in the study of nearly 10 million were discovered, and NONE of those tested positive for COVID-19.

December 23, 2020.

There was also a Danish study that showed that masks do not work. It is the largest and only (at the time) randomized control trial (RCT) on 6,000 people wearing masks and the results…

Masks DO NOT PROTECT YOU. Medical journals refused to publish it because it wasn't politically correct.

See www.mercola.com or Dr Mercola's past newsletters, June 6, 2021 Mask Propaganda Exposed, Brave Professor Speaks out.

Even liberal biased SNL did a comedy sketch in early 2022 called "COVID Dinner Discussion" on YouTube.

June 5, 2021-"13 Experts Rip COVID-19 Myths to Shreds"

To wear a mask or not should remain a person's choice and not a government mandate. This is what communism feels like. The government seeks to control you. Certainly, the elderly and high-risk individuals could have been advised to wear a mask and social distance and even self -quarantine if they feared getting it. The lockdown procedures caused more damage than we can even count, but in 2 sections we will discuss the collateral damage that the democrats caused. Now, lets find out where the flu went…

9.

FLU MISLABELED AS COVID-19

"When you're busy calling everything COVID-19 it makes sense why the flu numbers are down over 95%" - Facebook post, author unknown.

I hope your brain is questioning the probability of a 95% decline in flu incidence over a one year time period.

We have established that the (PCR) COVID test is NOT accurate even per the inventor of the test. So, plug that data into your brain and delete the old garbage and reprocess. Doctors were bullied and coerced into calling everything COVID. SCANDAL! There were multiple videos online by doctors who were asking the question why do they want me to call it COVID if it isn't. That is dishonest, right? The symptoms of flu are just about the same as COVID and the test does not differentiate them. Many people wrongly attributed the decline in flu to the mask wearing.

The reason that is not possible is that at the same time they were telling us that COVID was increasing. This was in the Fall of 2020 when the democrats were telling us that we should not spend time visiting our families at Thanksgiving because COVID was on the rise. Are you beginning to see how you were duped.

Here is some data on the recent flu fatality spike that did not warrant mask wearing for all by Fauci.

"Killer flu outbreak is to blame for a 42% spike in deaths in January after 64,000 people died-the highest number since records began." By Stephen Matthews for Mailonline. February 2018.

See also CDC stats for flu deaths in US from 2015 – 2020.

Using reverse psychology, perhaps there should be a class action law suit against Fauci for not saving the lives of those who died of the flu during the recent increase in flu deaths. According to his logic, masks would have saved lives.

December 26, 2020

From a Pharmacist thread on Twitter

"There's something very strange going on with this COVID thing. I have been a pharmacist for 43 years. It is well into flu season and I have not dispensed any Tamiflu, which is the most prescribed medication for the flu…it's well known that COVID tests give false positives. How many of these false positives are actually "the flu"? …I believe we are being played. YES, COVID

IS REAL. IT CAN BE DEADLY. We now have drug regimens to treat COVID effectively...I believe the COVID numbers are being skewed upward, on purpose to continue instilling fear and panic into people, for governments to continue with lockdowns, for more small businesses to be put out, for more people to commit suicide, or others...Total population control through fear.

You're slowly giving up your freedoms to a virus that has a 99.4% survival rate, according to the CDC. And the vaccine? Like I have told my customers all these years; don't be the first on your block to try anything new. They really don't know what they will find out in 6 months, one year, 5 years and longer, that can be attributed to the vaccine. It's way past time for people to take their heads out of their a** and start thinking for themselves." Harvey Staub

COVID IS "The New Flu"

10.

LOCKDOWN COLLATERAL DAMAGE

The lockdown strategy was falsely supported by the bogus number of cases created by the highly inaccurate PCR test for COVID and the bogus number of deaths due to COVID as they continue to count those dying with(comorbidity) or just possibly with COVID as opposed to actually dying from the disease in question. Let me say it again. Bamboozled! This is the biggest hoax ever to hit the planet, and if you know anything about how the devil works it is called deceit.

This section discusses how the lockdown efforts by the democrats actually caused more harm to Americans. Prior to August, 2020 even Dr Fauci said that continuing to close the country could cause irreparable damage. The CDC , prior to August 2020, backtracked on their initial claim that led governors to shut down their states and clarify that COVID actually does not spread readily on surfaces. Speaking of governors, Democrat Governor of New York, Andrew Cuomo, the nursing home killer, confirmed a recent health study showing that 70% of new infections actually originate at home (families sharing germs, how novel), thus making stay at home orders one of the most dangerous mandates currently in place.

As of August 2020, the CDC data showed that getting the flu shot (death rate of .6) is worse than COVID (death rate of .4) Should we stop advertising and giving the flu shot?

For the threat of COVID killing us, we have:

- added over 6 trillion to our debt

- laid off or furloughed 50 million workers

- gone from (record low) 3.5% to 14.7% unemployment.

- Crippled the petroleum industry.

- Ruined the tourism industry

- Bankrupted the service industry.

- Caused an impending meat crisis.

- Threatened, fined and arrested church leaders.

- Exacerbated mental health conditions.

- Shut down schools and colleges interfering with the education of millions.

- Increased suicide rates higher than COVID deaths.

- Delayed surgeries and treatments for serious conditions.

- Infringed on countless important civil liberties.

- Placed 300 million Americans on house arrest, where they were actually more likely to spread the virus to each other.

Are you one of those people who pointed the finger at others for not doing their part to keep others safe? Really, now?

Watch Megyn Kelly's segment called "The Truth: About COVID Hysteria Harming Our Kids"

Do you remember when all of the politicians and bureaucrats like Dr Brix told us not to travel and visit with our families, and then they went and visited their families. That is called hypocrisy and poor leadership and just plain dishonesty on the part of the democrats in office. Most of the Red states (run by republican governors) did much less locking down. Most Blue states (economically paralyzed by faulty democratic policies) did much more locking down. Looking at a graph of hospitalizations due to COVID per capita, California, the queen of the blue states has more than Florida, the red state and home of low taxes.

Incidentally, have you heard about the massive number of people moving out of Blue states and even Blue cities where things are poorly run and people don't feel safe with socialist democrat idiot ideas like defunding police. What sane mind would think that could help anything? It's SOCIALISM, people! Wakey, wakey!

For more information on the Collateral Damage caused by COVID, read the chapters entitled "Collateral Damage" and "Did Other Countries Fare Better-Sweden as a Role Model?" in the book Corona False Alarm.

11.

A POLITICAL VIRUS: RED STATES VS. BLUE STATES

A Red state is one that is run by a Republican governor and a Blue state is very sad because they have a Democrat governor. You learn that it is a very political virus when you see that the Red vs. Blue responses were very different and it should not be that way!

At one point in time, 26 Red states were open and 24 Blue states stayed shut.

This is so much more than "the election infection" and "the new flu"...

I want you to go to the following website and just review the fundamental differences between Republicans and Democrats on major issues:

www.diffen.com and plug in Democrats vs. Republicans

Big Picture: Democrats favored the lockdown strategy and it not only did not work to help save lives effectively, but it also damaged American lives in multiple ways to 6 feet under for suicide victims. Yes, they were victims of socialist democrats faulty ideology.

I am looking at a side by side comparison between Republican Governor of Florida, Ron DeSantis, and Democrat Governor of New York, Andrew Cuomo. Both states have approximately 20 million residents. FL has 0%tax rate and NY has an 8% tax rate. Time to move South! The FL budget is balanced and the NY Democrat is in debt. The number of COVID cases and deaths is about 10 times higher in NY than FL and on the surface those stats look really bad in NY, but when you consider statistical probability and the fact that this virus has reached pretty much around the globe you should question the accuracy of the data. We know that Gov. Cuomo managed it poorly. It goes back to the PCR test not being accurate and the cause of death often not being the virus, but other health problems that the person had.

Here is a summary of a few thoughtful insights from Trey Gowdy, former U.S. Representative from SC

"I'm not saying that COVID-19 isn't real...But pay attention folks, there is much more going on here than what meets the eye....

But there is something larger going on here driving this sudden outbreak right after Trump beats an impeachment attempt. Especially the fact that it, coronavirus, originated in China who we are in a global trade war with; brought on by Trump. Let's not forget Biden's back door deals with China as well. China does NOT want 4 more years of Trump either...

This is the perfect fascist playbook. Control the population with fear mongering and panic, control the media, spread propaganda and disarm the population."

Synopsis: Trump had the guts to stand up to China and punished them financially in our trade war.

Biden and other democrats have cozied up with the communists.

Fauci, a democrat, sent US dollars illegally to the Wuhan Institute of Virology to do "gain of function " research on this specific coronavirus that somehow (artificially) became able to not just infect bats but humans too and because it was new and for other reasons it became very contagious, but it was not highly lethal as some other viruses, so they used a bogus test to boost the case numbers and lied about the actual cause of death in many, many cases.

I say that he sent the money illegally because the US had banned this type of research, so he relayed the money through a third party, EcoHealth Alliance. Recently, he lied under oath during hearings conducted by Senator Kennedy of Alabama and then by Senator Rand Paul (who is an MD) from Kentucky.

12.

VOTING FRAUD RAMPANT

First, it was the Russian Collusion hoax and we learned that Joe Biden via his son, Hunter Biden, was actually receiving millions of dollars from Burisma. See the Hunter Biden laptop story.

Then, it was the bogus impeachment attempt. As I said, politics is dirty business. That, at the very least, was used to discredit our President even if the Left knew that they had no basis for the charges. You could say that "the gloves had come off" at this time.

Then, the coronavirus was released. Consider that Bill Gates hosted a coronavirus preparedness summit called Event 201 at The World Economic Forum in NY in 2019 shortly BEFORE the coronavirus got out of the lab. Could it have been an accident if these known perpetrators were involved prior to its release on mankind???

One reason that I am sooo upset is that I had a friend tell me in March 2020 that he had heard the radical Left Democrats were using the coronavirus to push the election process toward mail in ballots because it is easier for them to cheat on the vote count.

(See 2000 Mules, by Dinesh D'Souza)

In spite of ALL of this foul play, President Trump still won the election and there is ample evidence of this that has been squashed. Most commonly, the incumbent wins, but that is not my basis, but rather what fueled the Left to everything in their power with tremendous assistance from the liberal biased left wing mainstream media and social media.

IF you want the truth on what happened with the voting fraud the two main sources, I would point you to, IF you can "handle the truth", the entire speech by President Trump on 01-06-2021 at the "Stop the Steal" rally after seeking the courts to correct this injustice. Our very democracy is at stake if we cannot hold legitimate elections. You will also realize by watching him that HE DID NOT INCITE the violence that took place at the Capital. That is just how the Left wing media spun it along with the second attempt to impeach him with one week in his term which was to assure that he could not run again in the future.

The other source is two videos called "Absolute Proof" and "Absolute Interference" by Mike Lindell and this has gotten much attention and many views. Expect to find them not on Google owned YouTube, but on www.brighteon.com, where you can find truth telling banned videos.

No one has been able to give me a plausible explanation for why the vote counting was halted in only the battleground states on the night of the election. The real reason is that the Democrats had to know how much they needed to cheat by and then they made it happen. Dominion Voting Systems Corp. and Smartmatic are being challenged as to the accuracy of their voting systems. Who makes the decision on which company gets the job? Local governments do and not the Feds.

In Pennsylvania, 1.8 million mail-in ballots were sent out. 1.4 million were officially returned, yet somehow 2 million mail in ballots were somehow counted in total.

Facebook post-"Time to come clean. I work for Wayne County, MI and I threw out every Trump ballot I saw. Tens of thousands of them, and so did my coworkers. I regret nothing. From Kiel Fauxton

Have you studied the Electoral College vote map for the 2020 Presidential Election. A "swing state" is another name for a "battleground state" pretty much means that it is hotly contested and very close in the vote count. They include Arizona, Nevada, Pennsylvania, Wisconsin, Michigan and Georgia. One thing that most of them have in common is at least one large city where it is more possible of vote dumping. Get it? So, we paused the vote counting in the middle of the night to determine what the count was and then cheated by the number or more to win.

"We are not just talking about fraudulent voting acts. What we are talking about is TREASON! When you coordinate six to ten states, using cyber warfare to change the outcome, these are TREASONOUS acts."

-Trey Gowdy – U.S. Representative from SC

If just 3 of the bigger states that were wrongly awarded to Biden were restored to Trump, then we would be keeping America Great. Instead, look honestly at the downward spiral we are in with this socialist takeover. It needs to be reversed. Even though this has never happened before. The wrong needs to be righted ASAP.

Do you think Americans were justified in protesting the steal of the election? Do you know that the January 6, 2021 (Electoral College Vote Day) violence was not all Trumpsters. Are you aware that President Trump ordered Pelosi to beef up the security for the Electoral College process and she refused. Do you know that some of the same people from Antifa and BLM riots were also in pictures at the Capital breach. Are you aware of the proceedings that were going on and got halted and derailed due to this violence. As it turns out, Senators and Representatives from the "swing" states were objecting to the voting fraud that had occurred. This has rarely happened in past elections, but the evidence was overwhelming. Vice President, Mike Pence, presided over the Electoral College process to approve or challenge the integrity of the vote count. The State of Arizona had voiced their discontent with the vote count and there was to be a debate for up to 2 hours on each state contesting the vote count. The violence caused them to adjourn temporarily and when they returned Mike

Pence essentially just approved the vote. Was he paid off? Was he threatened? Who knows. The violence had a net effect favoring the democrats as it stopped the normal process of checking the system's accuracy.

Now, true democracy is in question in these great United States of America. The Democrats are trying to push a bill through called HR1 (aka-For the People Act) and it would move elections from state control to their federal control and like Venezuela we will go down the tubes with the failed system of socialism. Sad!

Voting issues that need to be addressed:

Extent of early voting, mail in voting, automatic and same-day voting registration, voter ID laws and ballot drop boxes.

Regarding the Democrats refusal to require ID to vote and Democrats policy on border control, which is currently a crisis of epic proportions for many reasons…have you put 2 and 2 together to realize they are OK with letting illegals into the country, give them free stuff and get their votes. Is that lack of ethics OK with you?

Who hires the vote counting software companies? The current company and way of doing this must change.

RESOURCE: Watch the documentary, 2000 Mules, by Dinesh D'Souza. It reveals the democrats massive voting fraud.

On January 6…This was the day that both houses of Congress met to potentially certify the election. Many Americans knew about the shenanigans that had taken place, but many of my readers may have been clueless about it due to regular viewing of the liberal left wing main stream media. Congress was to hear the complaints from the representatives of states alleging voter fraud on a massive level. Many patriotic Americans travelled to Washington to see if justice would be carried out. The media has framed the protests on January 6 as a violent insurrection, and conducted a circus like hearing. This should not be called a hearing, but rather a "smearing". A true hearing would listen fairly to both sides. Did you actually watch President Trump's speech on 01/06/2021? I did. He recounts the multiple reports of voter fraud in many states. He encourages action, but he does not incite violence.

By the way, how many people died that day and who was it that shot that unarmed woman? Compare to the previous Summer of violence funded by George Soros. Do you really think that people just randomly decided to go to these cities and burn everything down while the CNN reporter calls it a "peaceful protest"? So, how many people died in these riots? How many businesses were trashed?

That paragraph was to draw a comparison to the leftist sponsored riots and the patriots who were protesting the voter fraud as it robs us of our democracy. The states alleging voter fraud were to have a certain amount of time to protest the vote count and present their case. The representatives from Arizona entered their complaint before the interruption, and then they just went ahead and certified the election. The Electoral College system failed. Regarding the Capital building breech, look into a man named

Ray Epps. He was recorded on video wearing a red MAGA hat and instructing the protestors to go in the building. He was not apprehended. Could he have been a plant to cause a stir? There are also videos of Capital Police taking down the barricades so that protestors could rush in. Also, it is reported that President Trump instructed the then Speaker of the House, Nancy Pelosi , to fortify with more troops, but she refused.

On Mike Pence…Was he paid to swiftly certify the election? Was he threatened? I am of the opinion that they should have resumed the proceedings after the interruption. They should have allowed each state to testify and register their complaints of massive voter fraud. Then, proper forensic recounts should have been done in the "swing states" complaining of the voter fraud. I/ we do not know if President Trump had enough votes to win or not, but the democratic process must be upheld. Look at what we got!

The voting machines must not be connected to the internet. This opens the door to more voter fraud as was discussed in the videos put out by Mike Lindell such as "Absolute Proof" and "Absolute Interference".

2020 Election results tampering? Because January 6, 2021 became such a big event and the media coverage of everything related to it has been biased I beg you to look at each of these: 1) Watch President Trump's entire speech on Jan. 6 at the "Stop the Steal" rally. I saw it during my lunch break and he did NOT incite violence. 2) Watch the "2000 Mules" documentary by Dinesh D'Souza about HOW ballot dumping was accomplished and where. 3) Watch Tucker Carlson (FOX) interview of Tony Bobulinski in Oct. of 2020. He was the Biden's ex-business partner involved with the treasonous influence peddling scheme for multiple millions of dollars prior to the election. IF this were not buried, the election results would have been different. 4) Watch the TV interview of computer repair shop owner, John Paul MacIsaac, who became the legal custodian of the infamous Hunter Biden laptop. Do you know what is on there? Did Hunter pay his taxes? 5) Watch the documentary videos "Absolute Proof", "Absolute Interference", and "Scientific Proof". So, in summary, they delayed the announcement of the winner of the election allowing time to see how much behind they were in key battleground states. Then, alegedly funded by Mr Zuckerberg, the necessary number of bogus ballots were dumped in critical precincts. Look closely at the data and you will understand why protestors went to Washington. The violence is not condoned. You also should dig deeper into Ray Epps involvement at Jan. 6 and ask why he did not get in trouble and other trespassers did.

13.

COVID-19 VACCINES KILL AND HARM

A vaccine is a small dose of the pathogen administered with the intent of triggering an immune response and developing immunity to the pathogen. A vaccine may be live, killed or attenuated(weakened). Another classification of viruses and hence their vaccine is that they may be DNA or RNA. This is a messenger-RNA vaccine, a category which has zero FDA approved vaccines and yes, that should concern you.

Consider that Moderna struck a deal with the US government for $1.5billion and NO clinical liability.

The following is excerpted from a letter written by Dr. Frank Shallenberger, MD and it was posted on Facebook in December 2020. He has been in practice since 1973 and I think he is a good source of information on this. He explains why the vaccine is unsafe.

"Dear Patients and Friends,

1. The COVID vaccines are mRNA vaccines. mRNA vaccines are a completely new type of vaccine. No mRNA vaccine has ever been licensed for human use before. In essence, we have absolutely no idea what to expect from this vaccine. We have no idea if it will be effective or safe.

2. Traditional vaccines simply introduce pieces of a virus to stimulate an immune reaction. The new mRNA vaccine is completely different. It actually injects (transfects) molecules of synthetic genetic material from non-human sources into our cells. Once in the cells, the genetic material interacts with our transfer RNA to make a foreign protein that supposedly teaches the body to destroy the virus being coded for. Note that these newly created proteins are not regulated by our own DNA, and are thus completely foreign to our What they are fully capable of doing is unknown, but we expect auto immune disorders to result.

3. The mRNA molecule is vulnerable to destruction. So, in order to protect the fragile mRNA strands while they are being inserted into our DNA they are coated with (polyethelene glycol) PEGlated lipid nanoparticles. This coating hides the mRNA from our immune system which ordinarily would kill any foreign material injected into the body. PEGylated lipid nanoparticles have been used in several different drugs for years. Because of their effect on immune system balance, several studies

have shown them to induce allergies and autoimmune disorders. Additionally, these nanoparticles have been shown to trigger their own immune reactions, and to cause liver damage.

4. ~other toxins including aluminum, mercury and possibly formaldehyde

5. Since viruses mutate frequently, the chance of any vaccine working for more than a year is unlikely. That is why the flu vaccine changes every year. It's a different strain. (ME-they have had since 1918 to end the flu with vaccines and that has not happened) It is the wrong strategy!

6. Absolutely no long-term safety studies were done...If you ever wanted to be a guinea pig for Big Pharma, now is your golden opportunity.

7. Many experts question whether the mRNA technology is ready for prime time...

8. Michal Linial, PhD. Is a Professor of Biochemistry and she stated" I won't be taking it (the mRNA vaccine) immediately-probably not for at least the coming year. We have to wait and see if it really works...

9. (paraphrase) many healthcare professionals are reluctant to take it because the side effects are unknown...

10. Since the death rate from COVID resumed to the normal flu death rate in early September 2020, the pandemic has been over since then. Therefore, at this point in time no vaccine is needed. The current scare

tactics regarding escalating cases is based on a PCR test that because it exceeds 34 amplifications has a 100% false positive rate unless it is performed between the 3rd and 5th day after the first day of symptoms. It is therefore 100% inaccurate in people with no symptoms. This is well established in the scientific literature.

11. The other reason that you don't need a vaccine for COVID-19 is that substantial herd immunity has already taken place in the US. This is the primary reason for the end of the pandemic.

12. Unfortunately, you can not completely trust what you hear from the media. They have consistently got it wrong for the past year. Since they are all supported by Big Pharma and other entities selling the COVID vaccines, they are not going to be fully forthcoming when it comes to mRNA vaccines. Every statement I have made here is fully backed by published scientific references.

13. I would be very interested to see verification that Bill and Melinda Gates with their entire family including grandchildren, Joe Biden and Dr Fauci and their families actually got the COVID vaccine.

Here is my bottom line. I would much rather get a COVID infection than get a COVID vaccine. There are plenty of effective therapeutics to treat it."

Slightly paraphrased from Frank Shallenberger, MD

Can anyone explain to me why we would put our trust in a company, Pfizer, that has been sued 74 times for approximately $5 BILLION US DOLLARS since the year 2000??? Anybody?

I invite you to research on your own how much the other Big Pharma companies have been sued for. There is a reason why drugs are so expensive…their legal bills and court settlement payments are enormous. When will our society come to the realization that politicians are never going to fix our "health care crisis" and that Western medicine is a very flawed approach. (see Chapter 17 on this topic toward the end.)

By the way, I just saw a report that the vaccine is causing the coronavirus RNA to get into all of the organs of the individual. That sucks!

Here are some thoughtful questions posted on FB by a PhD. In December 2020.

Do you realize that this is NOT a normal vaccine?

Do you realize that this vaccine permanently and irreversibly changes your DNA?

Do you realize that a messenger RNA vaccine has never been licensed for use before?

Do you realize that if anything goes wrong, you have no recourse and probably no treatment to fix the damage done? This is in part due to it coming under (EUA) Emergency Use Authorization, which was improperly obtained.

Why did the BBC funded by Bill Gates peddle COVID propaganda?

Why is the biggest censorship campaign in force now?

Why is it that the "Great Reset" is being openly advertised yet people still deny it? (look it up)

Why is the mainstream media using celebs to further this propaganda and create fear?

Why are the fact check websites funded by the Big Tech elites?

There was a helpful "COVID-19 Vaccine Information Guide" published as a PDF file and I hope that you can find it still available at www.anchoredtotruth.com

Also, watch the documentary "Died Suddenly".

One key piece of information is that both AIDS and Ebola were quite nasty with a survival rate of only about 10-20% while the flu and COVID have about a 99% survival rate. Ponder that fact among the mass hysteria portrayed by the media daily.

Again, my heart goes out to anyone who lost a loved one to COVID. I am truly and deeply sorry.

You probably would not want to hear Dr Fauci say that it's about "the survival of the fittest". After reading this I hope you can see that HE IS RESPONSIBLE along with all of his coconspirators and there is a CLASS ACTION LAW SUIT underway.

I am now looking at a "Fact Sheet for Recipients and Care Givers". It includes the ingredients in the vaccine. Go to www. cdcvaccine.com

Essentially every vaccine that has ever been introduced to fight a virus has falsely been given the credit for slaying the virus. Look at graphs of timelines and death rates of infectious diseases and whenever you introduce a new germ to the immune systems of humans it takes a period of time to adapt. See "herd immunity" also. Then, vaccine is introduced as the disease has already declined in incidence. BUT, the CDC and the medics make billions on vaccines. Look at the drastic rise in the number of different vaccines recommended by your friendly MD. In 1962, there were 3, polio, smallpox and DTP (Diphtheria, Tetanus, Pertussis). Now, there are probably at least 33. I can't count that high. Many times, it is the other ingredients in the shot that are damaging such as mercury (thimerosal) used as a preservative causing autism for example. Did you ever look at the symptoms of autism and symptoms of mercury poisoning side by side. Mirror image.

Still trust your MD?

A quote from a person on FB…

"The belief that injecting synthetic chemicals made by habitually criminal companies who profit from perpetual disease somehow produces health is not only ridiculous and unproven-it is a foundational teaching of a dangerous religious cult that western medicine has become.

Does anyone know why Pfizer bought Arena Pharmaceuticals? Could it be that they make treatments for cardiovascular issues and autoimmune disorders (caused by the vax they just gave most Americans)? People are dying at alarming rates from blood clots and similar adverse effects.

A random post on Facebook said "Man encounters virus with a 99.7% recovery rate...and decides that permanently altering it's own DNA is the best course of action..." FEAR is a powerful weapon.

Dec 6, 2021 Yale Epidemiologist, Dr Harvey Risch: "COVID a Pandemic of Fear Manufactured by Authorities"

Nov. 12, 2021 WHO report that there have been 2,457,386 Adverse Drug Reactions from the COVID-19 vaccine. See www.vigiaccess.org

How many COVID vaccine deaths is acceptable to you? My number is ZERO. This is a prophylactic treatment of something that has a 99% survival rate so I see this as a gross violation of the Hippocratic Oath and those involved should be punished. The Hippocratic Oath is the oath that doctors take which basically says "first of all, do no harm"

CNN began reporting December 8, 2020 that we could expect some deaths. Reporter, Paul Joseph Watson. Coronavirus-CNN: "Don't be Alarmed" if People Start Dying After Taking the Vaccine- "That won't necessarily have anything to do with the vaccine." Make sure that you get the media's perspective. They are not willing to truthfully report the number of cases and deaths from COVID (see PCR and comorbidity discussion), but they are willing to say that IF you die just after the vaccine that the deadly vaccine did not cause the death.

This just in…as of November 2022, birth rates in Australia are down by 70% since COVID-19 vaccines started. Yes. They engineered it to decrease the world population. Insidious! That is how the devil works.

ARE YOU AWAKE, YET???

Many Pharmaceutical companies are making the dangerous vaccine. Including, but not limited to: Pfizer, Moderna, Johnson & Johnson…

Jan. 2022-Pfizer CEO, Albert Bourla, states that their vaccine offers "limited , if any protection against contracting the current variants"

Oh, speaking of J & J, their vaccine was halted due to people dying from blood clots that it caused as of April 2021, but they were able to get it back on line by 04-25-2021. Hey, they have more people to kill.

Patrick Henry of 2020 said "Give me liberty or give me death!!!Unless there's a virus with a 99% recovery rate, in which case, strip me of my freedoms, my job, my constitutional rights and put me under house arrest."

Back to the fact that the average age of a person who died from/ with COVID in 2020 was about 80 and above the life expectancy…

why are they advocating that young people get it???Follow the money trail and the death trail. I know, it's really sick! I am just reporting the truth.

Here is some hard data on how dangerous the COVID vaccine is and you WILL NOT HEAR THIS ON CNN! In the first three months of 2020 giving out this "free" vaccine, they killed more Americans than all vaccines in America in the past 10 years.

IF this were the Republicans agenda, then it would be exposed on CNN and other mainstream liberal media, but it is not. ALL of these evil players are Demoncrats. You need to take action!

Have you heard of VAERS(Vaccine Adverse Event Reporting System)? It is part of the cdc.gov site. Keep in mind that the only death reports there are ones that someone took the effort to put it there. I have heard it estimated that only 1 in 100 deaths get reported on VAERS. Who knows? Then, I just watched a convincing video on that banned video site www.brighteon.com and I was sickened to learn that they are deleting death reports and replacing with adverse event reports where the person did not die. If that is not propaganda, then I do not know what is.

Go to www.vaers.hhs.gov
Or www.cdc.gov/vaers

Thousands of deaths and hundreds of thousands of adverse reactions due to the vaccine. The CDC claims that all deaths are unrelated, reactions are mild and VAERS can't be trusted, yet they mandate that doctors report there.

Why don't these lives matter?

This stinks worse than chicken manure!

"The new coronavirus vaccine does not give lasting immunity.

It does not...

Eliminate the virus, prevent death, guarantee you won't get sick, prevent you from getting the virus, prevent you from spreading the virus to others, eliminate the need for masking (according to those who advocate masks), contribute to herd immunity.

Which all begs the question, what is it actually 95% effective at doing?"

BAMBOOZLED!

"There is absolutely no need for vaccines to extinguish the pandemic. I've never heard such nonsense talks about vaccines. You do not vaccinate people who aren't at risk from a disease. You also don't set about planning to vaccinate millions of fit and healthy people with a vaccine that hasn't been extensively tested on human subjects."

Dr. Michael Yeadon, FORMER VP and Chief Scientist of Pfizer.

Interesting quote!

Now, I am looking at a drawing of many people bowing down and worshipping the "Golden Calf" and it is labeled "vaccines". I wonder what happened to those people...

1Peter 5:8 -Be alert and of sober mind. Your enemy the devil prowls around like a roaring lion looking for someone to devour.

So, what is your favorite part of the new COVID-19 vaccine?

a. You can still spread the virus

b. Limited time of immunity

c. 10-15% reaction rate and unknown death rate

d. Increased HIV risk

e. Bell's Palsy

f. Anaphylaxis

g. NO manufacturer liability

h. Still have to wear a mask

i. Infertility

j. Auto-immune disease

k. ALL OF THE ABOVE

So, much later, Pfizer released their documents that revealed the vaccine does not have a 95% success rate as they said , but only a 12% effective rate. Liars for profit.

In C-SPAN covered hearing

Dr Fauci admits vaccines may contribute to autoimmune disorders. "There may be cross-reactivity between the peptides in the antigen in the vaccine and the peptides"…blah, blah blah says Mr Science. I call him Dr Evil.

See also Dr. Bryan Ardis video on the spike proteins makeup. It is called "Don't Drink the Water".

His discovery is that the coronavirus spike proteins, and the COVID vaccine, and the drug Remdesivir (the drug of choice to "treat" COVID) ALL have the same basic chemical makeup.

Fauci DOES NOT care about you.

There is a spiritual battle almost the size of Armageddon going on here and I don't think most people are getting it.

The Fauci emails were just released.

What in the world is a health bureaucrat doing communicating with a Big Tech giant, Zuckerberg of Facebook??? Answer: conspiracy , fraud, treason.

As "2000 Mules" explains Zuckerberg used over $300 million of his own money to conduct the ballot dumping in the battleground states while the final count was delayed.

So, did the "informed Americans" have a right to be upset and protest the election results. By the way, I am told that many Americans only guilty of trespassing are STILL being held without good reason.

If you have a sense of humor, then you will appreciate this, but if you got the vax and you are upset now, you may not like it.

One lab rat says to the other "did you get the vaccine yet?" and the other responds, "no, they are still testing it on humans"

See article by Lorenz Duchamps, <u>Israel, One of Most Vaccinated Countries in the World, Sets New COVID-19 Case Record</u>

And <u>Unvaccinated Have Lower COVID-19 Case,</u> Hospitalization, and Death Rates Than the Fully <u>Vaxxed,</u> by Julian Conradson. Jan. 23, 2022

You should be getting ticked off, but don't get mad at me. Turn your wrath on the perpetrators. The list is coming up in another section. I call them "Team Apocalypse"

Here are some other really good resources on this vaccine topic:

<u>www.vernoncoleman.com</u> and try .org
<u>www.mercola.com</u>

see 35 min. video interview with Dr Peter McCullough, MD

"Government Scrubs Stats on Vaccine Related Deaths"

Book, <u>Corona False Alarm , pages 99-116 .</u>

Book, <u>Unreported Truths about COVID-19 and Lockdowns.</u> Part 4: Vaccines.

Website article- <u>https://articles.mercola.com</u>

<u>Inventor of mRNA Vaccine Interviewed about Injection Dangers.</u>

Thought question: who owns the vaccine patents?

What is the money trail not only on the vax, but the entire scandal?

Antivaxxers are looked upon with disdain by the sheep who thought it was OK to put this toxic gene therapy experiment into their body. Again, if you did not "press pause" at the beginning of reading this, then you may get very upset. Nobody likes to admit they were wrong or even "eat crow" as the expression goes. The information I have presented here is overwhelming as it exposes the biggest scandal to ever hit planet earth. Please read it ALL. Plug the new correct data into your brain and reprocess. Take necessary actions.

Do you understand now why they want you to get multiple booster shots? Still think the same way?

Here is another video to watch. It not only exposes the corruption of "Big Pharma", but specifically iatrogenesis stats and the scam of statin drugs. Watch Tucker Carlson Today on Fox Nation. "Tucker Carlson interviews Dr. Aseem Malhotra on the corruption of medicine by Big Pharma."

14.

THE MAINSTREAM MEDIA'S AND SOCIAL MEDIA'S (AKA-BIG TECH'S) ROLE

Journalism may be defined as the production and distribution of reports on current events based on facts and supported with proof or evidence. (Wikipedia)

I see very little true journalism from the mainstream media especially on the topic of politics. It seemed that they spent about 90% of their air time during President Trump's term bashing him daily. The mainstream media has been the democrat's bullhorn for a good while now. Sadly, as the party has turned more and more toward socialism in recent years the media has stuck with them. Are you able to see through the bias as you watch? Do you ever get a counter balance to your news intake by watching conservative news reports as well? Observe the difference in spin and how much time is spent on certain topics and what gets left out. During the news what industry pays them for advertising slots more than any other? Big Pharma. Do you ever get tired of being instructed to ask your doctor for this chemical to put into your body? Do you ever get tired of them saying at the end of the ad "could cause death"? Remember the Hippocratic Oath in "health care"?

Is the world ruled by a small group of hyper-wealthy psychopaths? NO WAY. It would have been on the news, which is owned by that small group. (get it?)

Here, I am exercising my First Amendment right to free speech to speak my mind. You may not agree with everything I say, but I am sure I have made you think. Censorship has run rampant on social media especially leading up to the 2020 election and beyond. That is a breach of our first Amendment rights. Politicians are trying to right that wrong, but it is a difficult fight when they don't want to do right. Some of these companies are just too big. In the past they split Bell and Microsoft. It is past time to split these tech giants.

Most of the "fact checking" is really just them allowing what they want to be heard. Do not think for one minute that these "fact checkers" are the authority. They are owned by the big tech company.

'Who pays the vaccine "fact checkers"?

Factcheck.org is funded by a foundation that holds over $1.8 billion of stock in a Vaccine Company.

The Robert Wood Johnson Foundation is run by former director of the CDC, Richard Besser.

Nearly 15% of the foundation's assets are Johnson & Johnson stock.'-FB post

Q.) Do you really think that factcheck.org is an unbiased source of vaccine information?

The Law: Section 230 of the Communications Decency Act passed in 1996 protects big Tech from being sued for the content users put on their sites. I do not think it would be fair either. What about all of the foul language and the underaged people who may read that. Let's require algorithms that prevent certain profane words from ever appearing. I am offended by that. One of the 10 Commandments is "thou shalt not swear", and , in fact, they are the basis of our justice system, which is being dismantled. That's another downside to the socialist takeover.

Have you ever been put in "Facebook jail"?

Twitter permanently banned President Trump on the night of the election 2020. How about that free speech?

How can you tell when the truth is being told?

    -when Facebook blocks it…

-Twitter deletes it…

-Google hides it…

-YouTube bans it…

-Leftists forbid it…

-and media brands it a Conspiracy Theory.

My momma taught me to always tell the truth.

15.

MARXISM, SOCIALISM AND COMMUNISM IN AMERICA

Circa 1850 Karl Marx and Friedrich Engels, two German philosophers, were credited with developing the ideas we call Marxism, which is the basis for Socialism and Communism. There is just a subtle difference between the latter two. It is very ideological, but I do not think people living under this system of government have ever been truly happy. It has failed most everywhere it has been attempted. These three -isms oppose capitalism (aka-Keynesian economics) saying that it oppresses the working class. Rather than me defining these 3 -isms, I want you to look them up. Can you tell the difference between socialism and communism? They both fail.

Consider that the most robust economy the world has ever known was under President Trump and the democrats are destroying it!

The democrat party of today is not the same as it was 20 years ago. It has been hijacked by radical left wingers who are bent on destroying the America you and I know. Sadly, our educational institutions are pushing this garbage. Do you remember the "Cold War" and the fall of communism in Europe and Asia? It fell because it is a flawed system.

Another case in point, Hugo Chavez took office in 1999 in Venezuela. A country rich with oil has been run into the ground by this flawed system. The people there say that first they came for our guns. I fear that if they try that here, it will be a bloody mess.

Capitalism IS what helped to make America Great. Trump, with his business savvy, and not "on the take" as many politicians are, executed policies that allowed our economy to thrive. In fact, President Trump's economy had more black's employed than Obama's. So, who should the black vote go to? The party that promises free everything, yet limits the earning potential or the party that knows how to create jobs and grow the economy, and allow each individual the chance to thrive.

I wonder if most blacks know that it was the <u>Democrat</u> President Andrew Jackson who was involved with the initial taking of slaves circa 1830s and it was the <u>Republican</u> Abe Lincoln who freed the slaves. Do they know that the <u>KKK</u> was primarily made up of <u>Democrat</u>s?

Go watch all documentaries by Dinesh D'souza.

You may have noticed that I used the term "blacks" and not "African Americans". I do not subscribe to the political correctness doctrine. Many blacks are not from Africa. It is a race classification and I do not view blacks as lesser than whites. I am not a racist. I have many friends who are black. My code of conduct comes from the Bible, which says that God is not a "respecter of persons" so nor should I. Also, I agree with Rev. Martin Luther King in that we should judge people based on their character. My prayer is that the black community gets the 70% birthrate out of wedlock statistic way down as it is a fact that children NEED both parents involved in the nurturing process.

The democrats are trying to get your vote by promising "free stuff" and that is a principle of socialism that just does not work. Did you ever hear the saying "you don't get something for nothing"?

A good book for you to read is <u>Live Free of Die</u> by Sean Hannity.

Learn the term Progressivism. It is not good for America!

There is actually a book called "In Their Own Words-The Democratic Party's Push for a Communist America"

Wheeler has 5 Qs for Democrats:

1. What is the difference between socialism and democratic socialism?
2. Where has socialism ever worked?
3. Who pays for the free stuff?
4. What stops democratic socialism from turning into full socialism?
5. 5-Why would we want that here???

16.

MEET TEAM APOCALYPSE

The following people and groups should be investigated further for their role in the Coronavirus Scandal and the election fraud which is ultimately bankrupting America. Some are ring leaders in this circus of death and others were aiding and abetting.

The Chinese Communist Party, the Democrat Party, Dr Anthony Fauci, Ralph Baric, PhD (UNC) architect of the virus, Peter Daszak (EcoHealth Alliance), Bill Gates, George Soros, Bill and Hillary Clinton, Barack Obama, Joe and Hunter Biden, ALL of the liberal media companies for fraud, Big Tech companies including Facebook, run by Mark Zuckerberg, Twitter, run by Jack Dorsey, Google , WHO (World Health Organization), CDC (Center for Disease Control) {or should that be 'spread' rather than 'control'?}, The Author of the book, "COVID-19: The Great Reset"and Founder Klaus Schwab of WEF(World Economic

Forum- and The Davos Group), Big Pharma including Pfizer, Moderna, Johnson and Johnson and others, Neil Ferguson, patent owners of vaccines?

[The Deep State=The Illuminati=The Cabal]

You probably did not see this information on the media and that is because they would not report it. This is huge because it lends to the notion that this was all planned. In 2015, Bill Gates gave a "Ted Talk" entitled "The Next Outbreak? We're not Ready". He forewarned of a coming coronavirus and that he would be the savior in this coming pandemic. That is just chilling to me.

Then, in 2018, he ran a simulation that said it would kill 30 million in 6 months…

Then, in October 2019(note the timing), The Gates Foundation Hosted Event 201 at The World Economic Forum in NY (see also Davos Group and The Great Reset, please). "This was a high-level pandemic exercise that played out a novel coronavirus pandemic that could have potentially catastrophic consequences."

Do you still believe the lie that the virus came from the wet market in Wuhan or even that the leak was an accident???

See video on Patreon or Brighteon.com by Channel, Really Graceful. "An Alternative Opinion on why Bill and Melinda Gates are Really Getting Divorced."

See also on You Tube video 5:09 minutes by Journalist Saager Enjeti, "Epstein at Center of Bill, Melinda Gates Divorce.

Oh, then Gates resigned from his Microsoft board and diverted his energies to the COVID vaccine. This is a computer magnate who has billions of dollars. Why an interest in a vaccine?

Reminder that The Bill and Melinda Gates Foundation disguised as goodwill work gave 500,000 children in India a Polio vaccine and they got Polio and resulting paralysis.

There was a post on Facebook with Gates, Soros and Fauci pictured. The caption read" the same people who believe the earth is overpopulated say they can save your life with a vaccine"

Neil Ferguson was the British fellow who forecasted 500,000 deaths in UK due to COVID and 2 million deaths in U.S. due to COVID. Please remember to discard the statistics who died of comorbidities as that does NOT assess how lethal COVID is. (see p. 47 in Corona False Alarm)

Whoever released inmates during "pandemic". After all, weren't they safer in quarantine?

More information on the media can be found on National Pulse and Revolver.news. See also, p. 65 Corona False Alarm.

I want to paint a picture for you. Your TV is on playing the liberal slanted news. Just imagine two arms reaching out to you with a can of garbage. They open the lid to your skull and pour it into your brain. Now, you are brainwashed.

The WHO (World Health Organization), a division of the UN (United Nations) is reportedly run by the CCP (Chinese

Communist Party). Did you know that The Bill and Melinda Gates Foundation gives WHO more money than the U.S. does? Gates contributed 11.65% of their budget while the USA contributed only 7.85% of their budget and in fact Trump cut off money to them and Biden has restored it. Red vs. Blue again.

Recently, the WHO modified their definition of what a pandemic is by basically taking out the requirement to be lethal. It can just make people sick like having a cold and it can be defined as a "pandemic".

Remember that we said earlier that the WHO is the org behind diagnosis codes doctors use called ICD (International Classification of Disease) They initially created 2 codes for COVID: one was saying the patient definitely has COVID and the other saying that it could be COVID so let's just call it COVID. That falsely inflated the death toll.

Dr Anthony Fauci is the head of NIAID (National Institute of Allergy and Infectious Disease) which is a division of NIH (National Institutes of Health). Someone should expose his tax returns and actual income for the years 2019, 2020 and 2021. Does he really own or co-own any patent to the COVID vaccine? Did Senator Rand Paul subpoena for these items as he grilled him about the truth on the virus' origin?

In June 2021, the infamous "Fauci emails" were released via Buzzfeed and the Freedom of Information Act. They are very incriminating. Over 3,000 emails were released and they confirm that Fauci knew that "Gain of Function" research was being done in the lab and we know that he in fact funded it. Also, emails are between Fauci and Facebook CEO Mark Zuckerberg. Why?

We need to get some of the best forensic accountants busy on this.

Here is a post from Facebook and I just submit it for others to look into…

"The Chinese lab in Wuhan is owned by Glaxo!

Who, by chance, owns Pfizer!

Which, by chance, is managed by Black Rock Finance.

Who, by chance, manages the finances of the Open Foundation Company/Soros Foundation!

Which, by chance, serves the French AXA.

Coincidentally, he owns the German company, Winterthur.

Who, by chance, built the Chinese lab in Wuhan! Accidently bought by the German Allianz.

Which, incidentally, has Vanguard as a shareholder.

Which is a shareholder of Black Rock.

Which controls the central banks and manages about 1/3 of the global investment capital.

Which, incidentally is a major shareholder of Microsoft: Bill Gates, who happens to be a shareholder of Pfizer, who sells the COVID vaccine and he is a sponsor of the WHO."

Someone please look into the money trail for these "FREE" vaccines. From government to Big Pharma to patent owners???

Would somebody please investigate this? FBI?

Through the "pandemic" billionaires around the world gained $3.9 trillion while the working class lost it.

IF you are OK with this socialism creeping in do you really think they want to help you by giving you "free stuff"?

STOP thinking that people are basically good. The Bible teaches that we are born bad and in need of a savior. These people have skipped that step. Does that help you to understand? These are "very bad people" as President Trump said.

Satan is the thread that ties them all together.

Addendum of D words:

Devil	Dysfunction	Distress
Demon	Dust	Down
Death	Dirt	Distraught
Depression	Drugs	Diet
Disappointment	Drunk	Disaster
Discord	Drown	Diarrhea
Disease	Dogma	Deviant

Depleted	Denied	Defect
Deprived	Deficient	Deceit
Deleterious	Defecation	Democrat

Usually, when reading a list people notice the first and last items. Can you think of any others?

Look up videos on YouTube or Brighteon of Rep. Jim Jordan, Ohio grilling Fauci about his lies.

17.

EXPOSING
MEDICINE AND
PHARMACOLOGY
FAILURES

In the vaccine section I posed the question of why would we trust a pharmaceutical company like Pfizer, who has been sued 74 times since 2000 for approximately $5 BILLION to bring us out of the "pandemic"? A better question might be why should we even put our trust in MDs (Medical Doctors) and the practice of Medicine??? If you were aware that going to an MD is the third leading cause of death in America and it has been for a long time. It's called iatrogenic causes of death. Read on.

"Johns Hopkins study suggests medical errors are third-leading cause of death in U.S.- Physicians advocate for changes in how deaths are reported"

Yeah, let's just sweep that truth under the rug.

IATROGENIC DISEASE

The term iatrogenic is defined as "induced in a patient by a physician's activity, manner, or therapy. It is used, especially, to pertain to a complication of treatment." This is not just patient overdosing. The biggest subcategory is "non-error, negative effects of drugs".

Remember when I showed that the CDC keeps track of how many Americans die each year and from what cause? Curiously, they do not have a category there for iatrogenic death, but the numbers typically range from 230,000 to 284,000. You must go research how many Americans died at the hand of the MDs (Iatrogenic Disease) and plug that number in typically just below heart disease and cancer to come in third place. If you knew how many new drugs the FDA has approved you might think they are striving to take over #1.

This is NOT breaking news talking about Iatrogenic Disease and how MDs (Medical Doctors) routinely kill people and get away with it. Many other journals, institutions and newspapers have written on it in the past including JAMA (Journal of the American Medical Association), Harvard U., CDC (Centers for Disease Control), BMJ (British Medical Journal), The Lancet, New England Journal of Medicine, New York Times, Washington

Post, CNN, US News and World Reports. Someone needs to get the word out because this is not common knowledge, but it should be. Americans deserve to know the TRUTH.

Here is a chart of average numbers of iatrogenic deaths by category per year…(these are approximate)

DEATHS	CAUSE
106,000	Non-error, negative effects of drugs
80,000	Infections in hospitals
45,000	Other errors in hospitals
12,000	Unnecessary surgery
7,000	Medication errors in hospitals
250,000	Total deaths per year from iatrogenic causes

The WHO (World Health Organization) keeps stats on the major countries' health care performance. You would think that the U.S. would be #1 in all categories because we are the wealthiest nation on the planet (for now). Actually, we are near the bottom in most categories. But we consume more pharmaceutical drugs by far than any other country. Precisely the reason…drugs often don't enrich the health of the patient, but they do enrich the bank accounts of the MDs and Big Pharma.

THE OPIOID EPIDEMIC

This is a problem you probably have heard about. I once saw a statistical illustration stating that you could take the number of opioid fatalities in just one year, 2017, and that would be more than the total number of U.S. fatalities in the Vietnam War and the Iraq War combined. The opioid crisis is a pharmaceutical problem and 60 Minutes has done segments on it. They are saying that the Mexican drug cartels are now bringing more Fentanyl across the border with the Democrats "open border" policy. Sure, come on in, get free stuff and bring COVID too. Just be sure to vote Democrat. No, you don't need ID. Who cares?

February 25, 2022- NPR- "4 US companies will pay $26 billion to settle claims they fueled the opioid crisis. They are Johnson & Johnson, AmerisourceBergen, Cardinal Health and McKesson. So, J & J has some catching up to do financially.

Biggest ever pharma lawsuits by settlement amount-ranking the top ten:

10. Amgen - $762 million
9. Bayer and J & J - $775 million
8. TAP Rx - $875 million
7. Merck - $950 million
6. Eli Lilly - $1.4 BILLION
5. Abbott Labs - $1.5 BILLION
4. Johnson & Johnson - $2.2 BILLION
3. Pfizer - $3.5 BILLION plus
2. Actos - $2.4 BILLION plus
1. Glaxo - $3 BILLION plus

WOW! Sorry if they are not in order. Each has a lawsuit meter that is running.

No wonder Rx. is sooo expensive. Flawed system!!!

The point here is that we put our faith in these people to help save us rom COVID, the disease with a 1% fatality rate. Making any sense, yet???

THE VIOXX/CELEBREX DEBACLE

You probably know that NSAID drugs like Ibuprofen are infamous for causing gastrointestinal problems and others. So, the researchers found a new type of drug called COX-2 Inhibitors to treat pain such as arthritis pain. Vioxx was made by Merck Pharmaceuticals and Celebrex was made by Pfizer Pharmaceuticals. Vioxx was on the market in 1999 and taken off the market in 2004. Just when it was bringing the company $2.5 BILLION /year it was discovered to have caused 88,000 to 140,000 case of serious heart disease. By 2006 there were over 10,000 cases and 190 class actions filed against Merck. In 2007, Merck agreed to settle up for $4.85 BILLION! It was 27,000 individual law suits.

So, Pfizer must have someone on the inside at the FDA. In spite of causing similar problems to patients, as the 2 drugs are in the same class, just made by different companies with slightly different chemical compounds, Pfizer was allowed to return Celebrex to the market with a "Black Box" label. That is when the label must say essentially that this could kill you. I just want to remind them and you of the Hippocratic Oath, which states 'First of all, DO NO HARM'

Drugs DO NOT create health. A healthy person does not take drugs. If you met a person who takes 10-20 medications, would you think of them as healthy or really unhealthy?

See also…

Wikipedia.org List of Withdrawn Drugs

ProCon.org FDA Approved Prescription

Drugs Later Pulled from the Market

The list is extensive!

So, how do you know that your drugs and combinations are safe?

FDA approval…time…FDA withdrawal.

> "The total number of prescriptions filled by all Americans has increased by 85 % over 2 decades, from 1997 to 2016, yet the U.S. population has only increased by 21%. In 1997, 2,416,064,220 pharmaceutical prescriptions and in 2016, 4,468,929,929 prescriptions were filled.
>
> -Consumer Reports

Speaking of Consumer Reports , they did a nice article called "Deadly Pain Pills". "Every day, 46 people die from legal pain pills." Not just opioids, but on down to Tylenol.

Even aspirin can cause Reye's Syndrome and kill a baby.

KEY POINT: PHARMACOLOGY GOT ITS START IN WITCHCRAFT

"One of the first duties of the physician is to educate the masses not to take medicine."

-William Osler (1849-1919)

Every drug that has been recalled by the FDA was first proven to be safe and effective when approved by the FDA. The FDA is looking out for the interests of Big Pharma. Do not expect them to recall the COVID vax because they got Emergency Use Authorization in their fraudulent manner. Remember that there were /are effective therapeutics and drugs for COVID.

Picture a white-haired gentleman...

"As a retired physician, I can honestly say that unless you are in a serious accident, your best chance of living to a ripe old age is to avoid doctors and hospitals...

Almost all drugs are toxic and are designed only to treat symptoms and not to cure anyone."

-Dr. Allan Greenberg, MD

He is on to something there. Actually, our health care system is very good at acute care and trauma care. It is very poor at treating chronic conditions and that makes up ~75% of visits. Some sound advice would be to seek out alternative health care providers

Maybe if my ideas here are spread to every American and across the country, we can begin to fix our broken health care system. People need to say no to Rx. and 'yes' to healthy lifestyle and health will change. Obamacare was a disaster. Some had their health insurance premiums skyrocket. They failed to force the medics to come down on their charges. If a person has heart disease or cancer, for example, the medical bills easily run into 6 figures. I do not claim to have all of the answers, but I have shown that drugs do not lead to health, but some are needed. There are better ways.

18.

CLASS ACTION LAW SUIT: FRAUD AND TREASON, PAY DAMAGES ($$$)

I have been saying for months that there should be a class action law suit. Well, it's here! Go to www.sorendreier.com 1,000 Lawyers and 10,000 Doctors Have Filed a Lawsuit for Violations of the Nuremberg Code "A large team of more than 1,000 lawyers and over 10,000 medical experts, led by Dr. Reiner Fuellmich, has initiated legal proceedings against the CDC, WHO and The Davos Group (WEF) for crimes against humanity.

Fuellmich and his team present the incorrect PCR test and the order for doctors to describe any comorbidity death as a COVID death- as fraud.

The PCR test was never designed to detect specific pathogens and is 100% inaccurate at 35 cycles. All PCR tests monitored by the CDC are set at 37-45 cycles. The CDC acknowledges that tests over 28 cycles are not allowed for a positive reliable result."

How many professional athletes have a case for being disqualified from competing with a positive PCR and no symptoms? Example-Jon Rahm was just DQed from the Memorial Golf Tournament with a positive test and no symptoms. This is preposterous!

Dr. Reiner Fuellmich is an attorney from Germany and he also has an office in California. He sued Deutsche Bank and separately Volkswagen for their diesel emissions fraud and won each time. He has initiated the suit against WHO, CDC and the Davos Group. I trust that the other evil participants named herein will also be sued civilly and criminally.

Some are saying that Anthony Stephen Fauci should be tried for:

Treason (18 U.S. Code 2381)

Misprision of Treason (18 U.S. Code 2382)

Seditious Conspiracy (18 U.S. Code 2384)

Crimes Against Humanity

See Nuremberg Code

Here are some excerpts from the damning "Fauci emails"

As explained by Jordan in the video clip above, the email igniting the frenzy was sent by Kristian Andersen, an evolutionary biologist in the United Kingdom. Received by Dr. Fauci at 10:32

pm on Jan. 31, 2020, the email was in response to one he first sent to Andersen roughly four hours earlier. Attached to the email was a ScienceMag article written by Jon Cohen titled *'Mining coronavirus genomes for clues to the outbreak's origins.'* The article examined conflicts over risky 'gain-of-function' experiments and outlined scientists' investigation of genomes to explain the origin of the virus. It also reviewed the investigative experiments carried out by Wuhan Institute of Virology Director Shi Zhengli and her partner Peter Daszak (EcoHealth Alliance) on thousands of bats along with the discovery of hundreds of new coronaviruses.

After touching on several hypotheses for the origin of the virus, the article declares, *"The viral sequences, most researchers say, also knock down the idea the pathogen came from a virology institute in Wuhan."* Despite that statement, Andersen—not convinced the article makes a solid case for an evolutionary origin of the virus— replied to Fauci, saying:

> *"The unusual features of the virus make up a really small part of the genome (<0.1%), so one has to look really closely at all the sequences to see that some of the features (potentially) look engineered."* Andersen continues, *"I should mention that after discussions earlier today, Eddie, Bob, Mike, and myself all find the genome **inconsistent with expectations from evolutionary theory.**"*

Fauci is holding the "smoking gun" and the ballistics match exactly. Next, at 12:29 am on Feb. 1, 2020, two hours after receiving Andersen's email, Dr. Fauci sent an email to his deputy, Hugh

Auchincloss, M.D, with whom he has worked for fifteen years. The 'subject line' read "IMPORTANT." The 'attachments line' read "Baric, Shi et al. – Nature medicine – SARS Gain of function. pdf." The short email stated, "It is essential that we speak this AM. Keep your cell phone on." Adding, "Read this paper as well as the email that I will forward to you now. You will have tasks today that must be done." The email immediately forwarded by Fauci was the ScienceMag article that prompted Andersen's observation that the virus was "inconsistent with expectations from evolutionary theory."

The Fauci emails hold the evidence and they have become public. He knew that there were medications like Hydroxychloroquine and Ivermectin that are very effective at treating COVID. He lied to get the Emergency Use Authorization whereby his Big Pharma buddies will have zero liability for all of the people IT is killing. So, how many wrongful death suits is that for Fauci and all of those co-conspirators.

I saw a FB post showing Fauci behind bars. "This is what our next "Lockdown" should look like.

"Cardiologist and Professor of Medicine Peter McCullough testified in Texas earlier this year. Dr. McCullough sees COVID patients and says 85% of COVID patients given multi-drug treatment plan recover from the disease with complete immunity."

Other references, see also-

www.prepareforchange.net
www.agrdailynews.com
www.alethonews.com
www.thewatchtowers.org
www.thehighwire.com   by Del Bigtree

19.

RESOURCES AND REFERENCES

This section is a list of resources and references including books, websites, videos, conservative news sources and more. I am not a writer, but I have done my best to give credit to my sources as well as I can. I hope you can appreciate that. Please dig into these resources and research things for yourself. Unplug from the liberal, left wing "fake news" with its radical agenda that is destroying America!

Books

Corona False Alarm? Facts and Figures, by Karina Reiss, PhD., and Sucharit Bhakdi, MD, 2020.

Unreported Truths about COVID-19 and Lockdowns, by Alex Berenson, 2020.

The Truth About COVID-19, by Dr. Joseph Mercola.

Plague of Corruption, by Judy Mikovits, 2020.

COVID Operation: What Happened, Why it Happened and What's Next, by Pam Popper, 2020.

Live Free or Die, by Sean Hannity, 2020.

The Truth About COVID-19, by Dr. Joseph Mercola.

Neither Safe Nor Effective: The Evidence Against The COVID Vaccines. By Dr. Colleen Huber.

The War on Ivermectin. By Dr. Pierre Kory.

The Wuhan Cover Up: How US Officials Conspired With the Chinese Military to Hide the Origins of COVID-19. By Robert F Kennedy.

End of America, by Naomi Wolfe, 2007.

The Real Anthony Fauci, by Robert Kennedy. 2021.

(This also became a film documentary in 2022.)

Videos

Remember, if it got banned, that means it is good and full of truth they do not want you to see. Go to www.brighteon.com for "banned videos". Also, remember that Google owns YouTube.

Highwire with Del Bigtree did a video interviewing Dr. Fleming, MD, PhD going into the details of genetic engineering done on the virus in the lab.

Highwire with Del Bigtree video interview of investigative reporter, Jeffery Jaxen, regarding the Fauci emails.

"Plandemic" a 20 min. documentary with Judy Mikovits, PhD. Exposing Fauci in May of 2020.

"Absolute Proof" and "Absolute Interference" and "Scientific Proof" by Mike Lindell regarding Election Fraud. Also, see his website www.frankspeech.com

Watch Killchain.

Watch video by Tucker Carlson "Why did they lie to us for so long?" on You Tube.

Multiple film documentaries by Dinesh D'Souza.

"2000 Mules" explains HOW voting fraud occurred.

"2016: Obama's America" on plans to destroy her.

Another brand new and chilling documentary you must watch is "Died Suddenly" by morticians who are seeing these bizarre blood clots only since COVID started.

YouTube video "Tucker Carlson interviews Dr. Aseem Malhota on the Corruption of Medicine by Big Pharma" discussion of vaccines, statins and more

YouTube video "Tucker Carlson interview with Tony Bobulinski" regarding the Hunter Biden laptop and the Biden crime family dealings. The FBI buried it and it swung the election.

Video by Reiner Fuellmich, MD, JD with guest Dr David Martin regarding patents obtained prior to the virus release. (Consider that! Could it have been naturally occurring?)

YouTube "2015 Ted Talk by Bill Gates" He warned us of a coming pandemic. Thanks for telling us what you were up to. By the way, Bill, why do you give more money to WHO than the US government???

I also wonder if Mr. Gates has invested any money in the Big Pharma companies that produced the gene therapy "vaccine".

Readers should also investigate what happened when the Bill and Melinda Gates foundation funded polio vaccines for approximately 500,000 children in India. He gave many of them polio identified with the same strand as in the vaccine. He was banned from the country! So, why did the liberal, left wing media in the US continue to have a computer billionaire on their news broadcasts posing as a doctor during the "pandemic"???

Readers should also investigate and consider Bill Gates relationship with Jeffrey Epstein.

Video in 2015, Peter Daszak, CEO of EcoHealth Alliance states that coronaviruses are rather easy to manipulate. Hmmmm.

YouTube video "The Biblical Response to the Great Reset" with Pastor Jack Hibbs and guest Charlie Kirk. He lists the 8 objectives of the WEF.

Readers should research and investigate the WEF (World Economic Forum) founded and headed by Klaus Schwab. Look into their political ideals. Who attended the Event 201 in October of 2019? What was the agenda? This was the "rehearsal for pandemic". In January 2023, they held their annual meeting in Davos, Switzerland, with approximately 2500 in attendance. Is there any correlation between their members and the originators of COVID or the Freemasons? Is there a tie to Satanism?

On Rumble, American Media Periscope, "The COVID Cover Up". Sean Morgan interviews author, Dr Andrew Huff who was formerly with EcoHealth Alliance. His book is "The Truth About Wuhan". Sean also interviews Edward Dowd about the death stats in the youth.

YouTube video "Viral: The Origin of COVID-19 by Jordan Peterson and guest Matt Ridley" Paraphrase: 2 main reasons we know it IS manmade. 1) Law of Probability-is it coincidence that it originated in Wuhan, China where there is a lab that specifically does gain of function research involving "The Bat Lady" and Ralph Baric and the workers there at the lab were the first to get sick. 2.) Many experts in the field of virology agree that the gene sequence on the spike protein is NOT naturally occurring and that it must have been engineered. (see also Dr Richard Fleming's work on this)

NOTE: Matt Ridley explains that the way they engineered the furin cleavage site allowed for increased transmission.

Reader, please research/Google "mRNA technology". Be advised that NO other mRNA vaccines have ever been approved.

Video "How do mRNA vaccines Work? Here's what you need to know" Please note that this was put out by Johns Hopkins and that they were in attendance at Event 201.

NOTE: the COVID vaccine does not include the coronavirus! It is only the spike protein. What if the vaccine was branded as being good for you, but it is actually bad for you? See myocarditis, blood clots and infertility data.

YouTube video "All Types of COVID-19 Vaccines, How they work, animation"

YouTube video-"Unvaccinated vs. Vaccinated Protection from COVID" by Dr. Been, MD. Q) How long does "protection" last? They want you to keep getting boosters because it does not work and it is poison!

Many people have had COVID more than once. Many people have had the flu more than once. The flu has been around since 1918. The flu vaccine does not work. Viruses mutate as they wish. It is a flawed idea that makes billions for Big Pharma. Did you ever consider the idea of fortifying your immune system against ALL germs rather than injecting poisons? Not nearly as much money can be made on supplements, etc. because there is no patent to give the seller exclusivity. Get it? Did you ever watch the show, "Shark Tank"? If a new product does not have a patent on it, then they often want nothing to do with it.

YouTube video-FOX News- "Newly Discovered Fauci emails say COVID looked potentially engineered" FOX reporter interviews Dr. Marc Siegel.

YouTube video-on Rising-"Robby Soave: Fauci's SECRET 7 Hour Testimony on Gain of Function Lab Leak." Notice the research paper on bat coronaviruses that Ralph Baric, PhD

(Professor of virology and Epidemiology at UNC-CH) and "The Bat Lady", the Chinese virology researcher published.

YouTube video-Journeyman.TV- "Perspectives on the Pandemic/ blood clots and Beyond. Episode 15. Dr Sucharit Bhakdi, MD 2/2021.

YouTube video-Mark Zuckerberg, founder and CEO of Facebook Congressional hearing. He admits that the FBI told him how to censor stuff before the 2020 Presidential Election. (in YouTube search window, just enter Mark Zuckerberg Congress). By the way, did you know that he spent over $300 million of his own money to conduct ballot dumping in key "Battleground" areas to swing the 2020 Presidential Election. For more on that be sure to watch "2000 Mules"

YouTube video-"X Factor Winner Reveals World Secret Religion" This one tied it all together for me. I realized that Satan was behind it all. Freemasons??? I thought they were just a nice civic group.

Websites

Totalityofevidence.com (click COVID timeline)
Brighteon.com (for banned videos)
Wikipedia.org (for general info w/ a liberal slant)
CDC.gov
CDC.gov/VAERS
WHO.int

AAPSonline.org

TheNewAmerica.com

Zerohedge.com

PragerU.com

Mercola.com

Bitchute.com

BuzzFeed.com

FOXNews.com

Revolver.news

CONSERVATIVE NEWS AND TALK SHOWS

FOX News-Tucker Carlson, Sean Hannity, Laura Ingraham, Jesse Watters, Judge Janine

Mike Huckabee…

NewsMax

AON

Epoch Times

Gateway Pundit

Bill O'Reilly

Glenn Beck

Steve Bannon- "War Room" on app Real America's Voice

Doug Ross, Weasel Zippers, Free Republic, Bad Blue, The Right Scoop, Lucianne, Instapundit, The Blaze, Memorandum, Hot Air, The Drudge Report

Top Conservative Columnists: Jonah Goldberg, Mark Steyn, Andrew Stiles, Victor David Hanson, Michelle Malkin, Thomas Sowell, Walter E. Williams, Ann Coulter, John Stossel…

Top Conservative News Sites: Redstate.com, Dailywire. com, Reason.com, The Washington Post.com, The Conservative Treehouse.com, Spectator.com, Just the News. com, MRC.org, NYPOST.com, OANN.com, DailyCaller. com, Americanthinker.com, PJMedia.com, Townhall. com, JudicialWatch.com, TheGatewayPundit.com, LibertyNation.com, Breitbart.com, TheFederalist.com, ConservativeNewsDirect.com, ConservativePlayList.com, Whatfinger.com, Rantingly.com, Rense.com, AllnewsPipeline. com, LibertyNation.com, TheWashingtonFree Beacon.com, NationalReview.com, TheBlaze.com, PJMedia.com, Twitchy. com, RedState.com, LifeSiteNews.com, TheFederalist.com,

Conservative Political Advocacy Groups:

American Conservative Union

American Family Assoc.

Americans for Prosperity

Citizens United

The Conservative Caucus

Eagle Forum

Family Research Council

Freedom Watch

Freedom Works

The Heritage Foundation

SPREAD THE WORD!

Join the Grass Roots effort.

Please HELP by:

* sharing the message/e-book in this book to the groups and individuals listed above.

* sharing the message/e-book to your network, friends and family

* review the book/e-book

20.

SUMMARY

The coronavirus (SARS-CoV-2) was definitely created in the Wuhan Institute of Virology with U.S. money that Dr. Anthony Fauci illegally and inappropriately sent there via EcoHealth Alliance (Peter Daszak). Mr. Daszak was recorded in a video pre COVID talking about how easy it is to genetically manipulate coronaviruses. One of the research developers was Ralph Baric, PhD (UNC). He actually wrote journal articles along with the "Bat Lady" of Wuhan. The virus was most likely released intentionally when you consider that Bill Gates conducted Event 201 at The World Economic Forum in NY. This was a "dressed rehearsal" for a coronavirus pandemic that he had previously forewarned us of. See the video documentary " The Real Dr. Anthony Fauci" by Robert F. Kennedy. Wuhan lab employees were the first to get sick. Do you think the Chinese would keep good records on this for an audit?

COVID tests (PCR) are very inaccurate with a very high number of false positives, which created a fraudulently inflated number of cases after the 'curve flattened'. This was reported daily by the complicit liberal biased mainstream media (aka- the fake news).

Not only were the case numbers fraudulently reported, so were the deaths due to COVID. Comorbidities are other serious health problems that the patient already had and then perhaps they got COVID and died or perhaps they actually got the flu and since the test does not discern between the two. Doctors were bullied into labeling everything as a COVID death. Of course, the crooks behind this gave them financial incentive and newly created diagnosis codes. $39,000 to hospitals for putting a patient on a ventilator and there is approx.. 80% chance of death after that. Heroic measures that are known not to work.

The treatment of COVID has been inappropriate. We could debate what is the best treatment approach, but I have shown that the medications Hydroxychloroquine and Ivermectin as well as monoclonal antibodies, Vitamin D and C and zinc all have been found to work well. So, there were other effective therapeutics all along and the Emergency Use Authorization for a very dangerous vaccine should never have been given.

Masks are not healthy nor are they effective per the AMA and even Dr Fauci was on record previously saying so. This is partly about control and partly about having a visible physical manifestation and associated fear factor to run up to the election fraud.

The flu (influenza virus) did not leave the planet during 2020. It was not the mask wearing that decreased the flu numbers by 95%. That is not statistically probable especially when COVID numbers were reported to be escalating. Again, the PCR test does not discern the two and the symptoms of both are about identical.

Lockdowns have been shown to be more harmful than any benefit they may have theoretically produced. Increased suicides, jobs lost, businesses lost, bankruptcies, increased national debt and resulting inflation and rising costs. This could have all been averted IF Fauci had just spoke the truth and said that the curve is flattened now, in June 2020, you can go back to work.

Remember that a friend told me in March 2020 that the dems were going to use COVID to skew the election and I thought… "huh? No way!…" Way!

The political connection has been discussed at length, but it concerns me to learn that this was not just "the election infection" and it is not just "the new flu"…it is being used to further the radical leftist liberal democrat agenda of implementing communism/socialism in these United States. They are doing it full speed ahead. Collision is coming! Are YOU awake, yet?

Many think that Trump WON the election in spite of all that the cheating democrats did. The election was stolen and they should have properly recounted the votes in some of the "swing" states. I suggest a proper recount in all of the states where massive democrat voting fraud took place. This has never happened before, but democracy and capitalism is being replaced with socialism and it is not good for America. This is a call for justice! NOT for violence.

The COVID-19 vaccine is not 'good' as the media reports. It killed more Americans in the first 3 months than ALL vaccines in America over 10 years. Think! Watch the documentary "Died Suddenly". This is supposed to be a prophylactic treatment to prevent getting it and IT IS KILLING PEOPLE! That is not OK. Zero of these deaths are OK with me. The VAERS system tracks how many adverse reactions and DEATHS get reported. Now, they are deleting death reports and replacing with adverse event reports. Fraud! Have you seen enough evidence that these people ARE trying to reduce the world population?

Key Point: COVID-19 vaccine AND Rx-Remdesivir both have the same chemical composition as the spike protein on the SARS CoV-2 virus. Let that sink in.

Serious adverse reactions due to the COVID-19 vaccines have become prevalent and include, but are not limited to auto immune diseases, myocarditis (often fatal), blood clots (often fatal), infertility and "long COVID".

Your democrat run government has poisoned you with an untested Emergency Use vaccine that is killing and harming countless numbers of people. Please watch the new documentary "Died Suddenly". Now, they are trying to require vaccine passports. Oh, this just in, the G-20 summit approved vaccine mandates for the next pandemic. This means you will not be permitted to travel freely. It is NOT about helping to protect us. It IS about controlling us. This is evidenced by the fact that the vax does not work.

The mainstream media and social media companies should be punished in the class action law suit that is underway.

Whenever you vote in the future, just remember that it was the democrats who brought you: this coronavirus and the poison COVID vaccine, masks, unemployment and suicides from the lockdown, censorship, socialism, vaccine passports, racial violence and Critical Race Theory(CRT) (a socialist ploy to divide us), increased national debt, inflation, lawlessness, border crisis, abortion , more taxes and much more evil.

ACTION STEPS:

+Get involved! Fight tyranny (legally).

+Reproduce the flyer on this website's home page and distribute it. Talk it up. We need a "grass roots" effort because the mainstream media will not pick this up.

www.coronavirusscandalexposed.com

@COVIDscaminfo on Twitter

+ NEVER vote for a democrat again. Doing so makes you an accomplice to murder (abortion is advocated by virtually every democrat politician)

+Seek out alternative health care providers and doctors.

+Unplug from the media, both mainstream and censored social media.

+Share this with the above listed groups and individuals.

INSTEAD OF CALLING THEM "CONSPIRACY THEORIES", WE SHOULD CALL THEM "SPOILER ALERTS"...

Please read Ephesians Chapter 6 and especially verses 12-13.

QUESTIONS to ponder and research:

Q) Why did Judy Mikovits get locked up?

A) watch the video "Plandemic"

Q) Why did the liberal main stream media lie and say that the virus came from a wet market in Wuhan?

A) They are the mouthpiece of the Democrat party. It is not journalism. It is propaganda with an agenda.

Q) How did Dr Kary Mullis, PhD., founder of the PCR test (aka-COVID test), actually die? He died just before the COVID outbreak. NOTE: Mullis hated Fauci because he misused the PCR test. Watch the video.

A) very suspicious

Q) why did Dr Fauci insist on using the PCR test as a standard to test for COVID, even though the founder of the test, Dr. Mullis, told him vehemently that the test is not specific to a certain virus. It only multiplies the sample. Why did the WHO set the number of cycles so high on these COVID tests?

A) Same answer for both. To increase the case count so the media could scare us daily.

Q) Why did a person dying WITH COVID become dying FROM COVID? Keep in mind that, sadly, people die every day and the average age of person dying from COVID in 2020 was about 80 years of age.

A) This was done to increase the death count to scare you more. Most died from comorbidities, that is they had other serious health problems and it was their time to go. Remember that the fatality rate for COVID is less than 1%, making it very similar to the flu.

Q) Keeping in mind that the flu has been around since 1918 and the flu vaccine is worthless, why didn't Fauci force us to wear masks in recent years as cases and deaths have risen significantly?

A) It was not an election year.

Q) How do you prove to someone that the COVID death stats were fudged?

A) Look at the CDC annual cause of death graphs. In a typical year about 2.8 million Americans die. COVID was a new cause of death in 2020. Some state that 350-500,000 Americans died in 2020 FROM COVID. The actual increase in deaths in 2020 was closer to 70,000. This is evidence that most people died of other causes and they were labeled as having COVID. Deceit!

Q) Since the fatality rate of COVID was only about 1%, like the flu, could it be that the "end game" was to get the jab into your arm?

A) Many think so. Look at the soaring numbers of myocarditis cases, blood clot deaths, and decreasing fertility rates.

Q) Since the coronavirus causes COVID, and vaccines usually have the germ in them, why does the COVID vax have the spike protein, but not the virus?

A) I am going to answer a Q with a Q...Why is the same chemical makeup in the spike protein and the jab and the drug? What is the world population?

Q) Why were Big Tech companies like Facebook, Twitter and Google all found to be involved in censorship of the truth?

A) Simple. They are in on it.

Q) Why did the WEF (World Economic Forum) along with bill Gates, host Event 201, a Pandemic Rehearsal, in NY on 10-18-2019 and then BOOM it happened? Who attended the meeting? Who has attended their meetings since? Is there any overlap in attendees there and on Epstein Island? Just asking.

Q) Why did the Democratic Biden Administration push for the unconstitutional vaccine mandate, which was disallowed by the courts?

A) Thoughts?

Q) Is there a connection between members of the Freemasons and the people behind the COVID scam?

Follow us on Twitter @COVIDscaminfo

www.ingramcontent.com/pod-product-compliance
Lightning Source LLC
Chambersburg PA
CBHW060240030426

42335CB00014B/1553